Healing Civil War Veterans *in* New York *and* Washington, D.C.

HEATHER M. BUTTS | *Foreword by Hugh F. Butts*

THE
History
PRESS

Published by The History Press
Charleston, SC
www.historypress.net

First published 2019

Manufactured in the United States

ISBN 9781625858900

Library of Congress Control Number: 2017958380

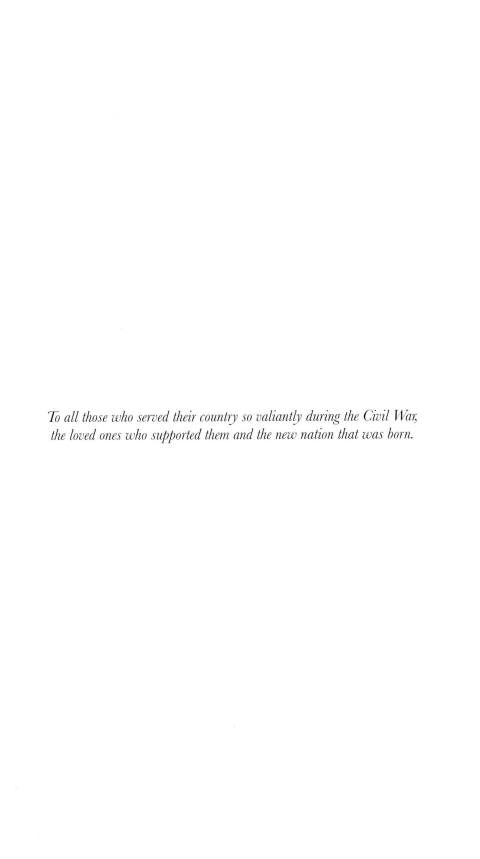

*To all those who served their country so valiantly during the Civil War,
the loved ones who supported them and the new nation that was born.*

CONTENTS

Foreword

It piqued Professor Heather Butts's interest in the topics of psychic pain and healing as she gained increasing knowledge about the problematic health and medical care issues relative to Americans of African descent, dating back to slavery. A further consideration for a book project drew perpetual concerns from those who questioned the amount of effort required. Butts did not deny her uncertainties, but was driven by the need to address a fundamental issue of human well-being and survival. This work tells an edifying story of initiative, responsibility, determination and empowerment. However daunting, pursuing the challenge became an unshakable commitment for Butts.

Her academic preparation, including completing her undergraduate/ graduate studies at Princeton, St. John's Law School, Harvard School of Public Health and Columbia University School of Education/Psychology, established a solid foundation for her research pursuits. Various work experiences, including the creation of a nonprofit program and engaging in hours of research on the organization made her well prepared for the task she undertook as the author of this literary work. It reflects a legal, physical, psychological, public health and educational focus, which offers an inspiring multidisciplinary orientation to her material.

Her study is complex. Professor Butts deserves scores of accolades for providing enlightenment regarding this momentous period in American history.

It came as a pleasant surprise when, in October 2016, I received a request from Professor Butts, my daughter, to once again write a foreword for a book she was writing. She discussed that some areas the book would focus on included symptoms of PTSD, coping mechanisms, treatment and a historical perspective of PTSD. I was eager to accept.

PTSD is descriptive of a specific symptomology that emerges in extreme trauma. The physical and mental effects include stress, depression and anxiety, among others. These responses can vary from individual to individual, but with increased realization, it has become clear that these responses are fairly typical. Stressors can be expressed by indirect contact with trauma. Symptom development is relative to exposure to trauma. People who exhibit blatant wartime contact have symptomology that is much more prominent than people at a considerable distance from the direct war. This disease can begin in a mild form and become elevated as time goes on, with or without increased exposure to the trauma itself. Healthcare workers can also experience PTSD during war; in some cases, the disorder can be subtle and in other cases fairly dramatic. Symptoms of PTSD begin mildly in most instances and gain intensity as time goes on, spreading from the nervous system so that at first a patient may complain of difficulty falling asleep, which is mild in intensity. With the non-passage of this symptom, patients may develop full-blown insomnia and difficulty sleeping. Traumatic dreams may disturb sleep and nightmares that are initially frightening become more traumatic with time, but especially regrettable is that many patients do not receive help because of a tendency to minimize their difficulties in the face of overwhelming trauma.

Professor Butts also examines the role between racism and trauma. The more we examine racism, the more we can test its intense reaction in people who are exposed. This symptomology begins in a mild form and increases over time. Slavery was an exaggeration of their original trauma, which may have been repressed. It can be just as traumatic as the secondary trauma of war and deserves exploration.

The book also deals with trauma of children during the war, particularly orphans. Any trauma, physical or mental, that affects children's lives is to be taken very seriously. Children can be more susceptible to the effects of trauma than older individuals because of their lack of complete formation and their inability to cope in the same manner as adults. They do not have the defenses that adults have, and for those whose parents have died, they do not have the parental presence for support. Plus, during the Civil War, society did not have the sensitivities to assist these children.

I found this a fascinating experience whereby my daughter is involved in exploring an area of research that is near and dear to me, trauma. I feel it creates a kinship for me to be involved in the book that seems natural and allows me to expand my thinking on the subject and expand my thoughts from her first book, *African American Medicine in Washington, D.C.* I am glad to travel this journey with her and the reader.

Many psychiatrists such as myself have been encouraged by the spread of interest in PTSD because it leads to more investment and more research that applies to the world at large, enabling investigators to feel their work is helpful in the broader scope of trauma research and solution.

The Civil War was a traumatic experience for man. Slavery had a widespread effect. It's important to write a book on PTSD and the Civil War—not only is it research that cannot be turned away from but undoubtedly this work will have a marked impact on the entire reader. It cannot be minimized. It should not be ignored. It has current public health, legal and medical implications. I am proud to be a part of this important and timely project.

—Hugh F. Butts, MD

PREFACE

The focus of this book will be the health and healthcare of Civil War participants in New York and Washington, D.C. The focus of the book is psychological trauma, post-traumatic stress disorder (PTSD) and recovery. The book's hypothesis is that many Civil War soldiers exhibited PTSD symptoms during the war and developed secondary healthcare issues, such as alcoholism, morphine addiction, trauma and physical challenges. These share a comorbidity with PTSD, and those affected used myriad ways and mechanisms to cope with that trauma. A clearer understanding of the physical impact of the war may have led to better healthcare outcomes postwar. The book will also review hospital facilities in New York and D.C. that cared for these individuals after the war.

I have had a long-standing interest in trauma, PTSD and healing after a traumatic event. My parents are both mental health professionals. My father is a psychoanalyst, and my mother is a psychiatric social worker. They were a wealth of information on various topics, including resiliency post-trauma. I was fortunate early in my academic life to author a paper with my father titled "Housing Bias and Post-Traumatic Stress Disorder." It was published in the late 1990s, and it was after its publication that I pursued examining trauma and healing around wartime. My first book, *African American Medicine in Washington, D.C.: Healing the Capital during the Civil War Era*, began that exploration, and this book continues that work.

The epilogue will go into more detail regarding modern-day implications of trauma and recovery. However, a brief note regarding this is warranted here. In the aftermath of the Civil War, many who fought and served during the war were expected to seamlessly return to their former lives. For many, especially those with physical and emotional wounds, this was impossible. My hope is that through examining how those suffering from trauma after the war coped, as well as the type of care they received, insight can be achieved for those ravaged by traumatic experiences in current times. Additionally, coping mechanisms for people in psychological pain are varied. We have all seen the ravages of the modern-day opioid epidemic and the many reasons why individuals become addicted to pain medications. Can we learn anything in modern times from the lessons of the Civil War era? Yes. This book will explore these lessons.

ACKNOWLEDGEMENTS

Many acknowledgements need to be given here. First, to my family, my mother, father and sisters, Sydney and Samantha, who stood by me from the inception of this book until its conclusion. I am extremely grateful to my loving family who fully supported my efforts. My mother, Clementine R. Butts, LCSW, was facilitator and problem solver to get the work done, and my father, Hugh F. Butts, MD, provided insightful consultation. My sisters, Sydney C. Butts, MD, FACS, never allowed me to compromise on my goal to achieve excellence, and Samantha F. Butts, MD, MSCE, established positive alternatives as a means with helping to maintain a balance in my life. My entire family has always modeled the kind of courage and valor that I hope I have conveyed through my writing this book.

Next, to my dear friends and proofreaders. Thank you to the amazing Phyllis Mathis and Anthony Antonucci, who gave feedback and encouraged me to progress and finish the text. And thanks to my professors and mentors at Princeton University, Harvard University, St. John's Law School and Columbia University, all of whom supported my work in different ways.

Of course, so much thanks goes to my amazing editor Banks Smither of The History Press. His patience and support were invaluable. He has been a consummate professional and positive presence during this endeavor.

Thank you to Elliot Gibbons and Jon Gibbons for providing me with an oasis to think, write and enjoy the sunshine. I couldn't have finished the book without you. To Councilmember Debi Rose of Staten Island and her amazing staff members, I love you all. Additionally, Deborah Marton, Alan Miller, Sarah Blas, Harriet Washington, Dr. David Rosenthal, Matthew and Kristen Costello, Andrew Smith Lewis and the Smith Lewis family, Sandra Smith, Michael Smith, the Whitmore-Turner family, Peter Carter, Anita Jones and family, Elise Jaffe, Cherryl Bailey, Michael Price, the Kirkland-Thomas family, Curtis Green, Sam Salant, Bill Grainer and the Grainer family, my friends at LIU Post, Columbia University, St. John's University, Nene Antonucci, Lexi Antonucci, Diana Dell, Carol Dingle, Miles and Lucy Gibbons, the Forty-Seventh Infantry reenactors, Dr. Turner Kitt, Von Barron and Joanna Barron.

A deep gratitude to Professor Margaret Turano for her constructive guidance and enduring assistance; to Cliff E. Barnes Esq., my astute Washingtonian mentor who advised about the timeliness of the book; Lu Willard and Stanley Hoffman began creating public interest in the book well ahead of its arrival; David A. Brockway maintained a listening ear, always ready to be an objective sounding board; Robert J. Ruben, MD, has greatly enhanced the quality of my life from early childhood; Cheryl Hill, who shared some interesting early history about members of her Washington family in the healthcare field; Alan Miller, MD, a wonderful mentor whose commitment to public health work inspired me to pursue that academic path; to my board and staff family at the Northside Center for Child Development—you inspire me daily with your commitment to helping others; Judith Nigro, Diana Dell, Carol Dingle, so many devoted extended family, friends at the Staten Island Greenbelt; my loyal Kew Forest family; and Dr. Frank Smith of the African American Civil War Memorial and Museum, who encouraged me to continue with my research. Finally, thank you to everyone at The History Press for their talent, patience and support.

I hope you enjoy this publication, which I believe has importance for all of us. My hope is that this inspires those who read it to delve even more deeply into this important piece of our country's story.

INTRODUCTION

Whether it is called shell shock or soldier's heart, experienced during the Civil War or the Vietnam War, the devastation that wartime trauma leaves in its wake is undeniable. Historical diaries of soldiers, nurses and physicians acutely speak to the horror and trauma individuals have suffered during wartime. The studies documenting the traumatic effects of combat on wartime participants are numerous.[1] Following on the heels of these studies[2] came the recognition that civilians, subject to certain stressors, seemed to display many of the same symptoms that wartime veterans exhibited. While many of these studies of civilians are insightful and instructive, they often raise still further questions for those in wartime situations regarding traumatic responses. What types of stressors are enough to induce post-traumatic stress in individuals?[3] Are individuals from different ethnic backgrounds apt to respond differently to different stressors? Are individuals who have suffered traumatic events in the past more primed to suffer post-traumatic stress disorder? What are the legal ramifications of PTSD?[4]

1

POST-TRAUMATIC STRESS
DISORDER OVERVIEW

EPIDEMIOLOGY AND PTSD

Epidemiology examines the rate at which a particular disease affects a distinct community, with the goal of determining the prevalence of the disease and developing a resolution to the problem. The evolution of PTSD as a formal disease has taken various turns. Accounts of railroad accidents of the late 1800s and early 1900s document "traumatic episodes" that workers experienced. PTSD occurs after an individual is confronted with an extreme stressor. As terms such as *soldier's heart*, *war neurosis* and *shell shock* entered the vernacular, a formalized concept of post-traumatic stress was born.[5] This formalization first appeared in the *Diagnostic and Statistical Manual of Mental Disorders* (DSM) in 1980.[6]

One controversy regarding retrospectively diagnosing PTSD is because it was not a recognized syndrome during the Civil War. According to Sarah Ford:

> [T]*he first mention of symptoms correlated with PTSD dates back three thousand years ago, four thousand years before it would be clinically recognized. Ancient Egyptian Hieroglyphics depicted the emotions and fears soldiers felt while in combat. The Greek historian Herodotus wrote in 480 B.C. of a Spartan soldier who was taken off the front lines due to his trembling and later took his own life in shame. In the seventeenth*

century, any disorder associated with depression or changes in personality was termed melancholy or nostalgia. Symptoms similar to PTSD were called Soldier's Heart and Da Costa Syndrome during the mid and late nineteenth century.[7]

Ford goes on to state that "[t]he catalyst for the recognition of PTSD was the outbreak of World War One. The Great War had some of the worst casualties in human history as a result of revolutionary weaponry that redefined warfare. The psychological effects of this war were often seen in the returning veterans as many experienced involuntary ticks and shook unaccountably. This later would be termed Shell Shock."[8]

Future chapters of this book will delve more deeply into the Civil War and specific PTSD triggers; however one issue that must be addressed is the weaponry used. While discussions of the Minié ball often focus on the physical aspect of the destructive nature of the projectile which was prone to shatter anything it encountered, the psychological devastation it wrought on its victims is undeniable.[9] According to author Sarah Ford, the railroad was a modernizing advancement in the wartime efforts, but it may also have been a part of the trauma experienced by participants. By not having to rely on horses as a mode of transportation, individuals had easier access to travel and soldiers saw more tragedy than ever before, thus affecting them on a broader psychological level:[10]

*Exposure to traumatic experiences has always been a part of the human condition. Attacks by saber tooth tigers or twenty-first century terrorists have likely led to similar psychological responses in survivors of such violence. Literary accounts offer the first descriptions of what we now call posttraumatic stress disorder (PTSD). For example, authors including Homer (*The Iliad*), William Shakespeare (*Henry IV), and Charles Dickens (*A Tale of Two Cities) *wrote about traumatic experiences and the symptoms that followed such events. The PTSD diagnosis has filled an important gap in psychiatry in that its cause was the result of an event the individual suffered, rather than a personal weakness. PTSD became a diagnosis with influence from a number of social movements, such as Veteran, feminist, and Holocaust survivor advocacy groups. Research about Veterans returning from combat was a critical piece to the creation of the diagnosis. War takes a physical and emotional toll on Service members, families, and their communities.*[11]

Early Attempts at a Medical Diagnosis

European descriptions of the psychological impact of railroad accidents added to the early understanding of trauma. Austrian physician Josef Leopold wrote about "nostalgia" among soldiers. For soldiers exposed to military trauma, reports of missing home, feeling sad, sleep problems and anxiety were not uncommon. These symptoms were a model of psychological injury post–Civil War. Another theory suggested a physical injury as the cause of symptoms. Rapid pulse, anxiety and difficulty breathing marked "soldier's heart" or "irritable heart." American physician Jacob Mendes Da Costa studied Civil War soldiers with these cardiac symptoms and described it as an overstimulation of the nervous system. The condition became known as "Da Costa's Syndrome." Soldiers frequently returned to battle after receiving various medications to deal with symptoms.[12]

According to the National Center for PTSD (NCPTSD):

> *Post-traumatic Stress Disorder, or PTSD, is a psychiatric disorder that can occur following the experience or witnessing of life-threatening events such as military combat, natural disasters, terrorist incidents, serious accidents, or violent personal assaults like rape. People who suffer from PTSD often relive the experience through nightmares and flashbacks, have difficulty sleeping and feel detached or estranged, and these symptoms can be severe enough and last long enough to significantly impair the person's daily life.*[13]

The NCPTSD fact sheet asserts that, besides the psychological component, PTSD has a biological component. PTSD can lead to disruptions of a person's interpersonal, professional and social life.[14] One characterization of a traumatic event, according to Yehuda, is its capacity to provoke "fear, helplessness or horror in response to the threat of injury or death."[15]

Hidalgo and Davidson state that in order for an individual's symptoms to qualify for the diagnosis of PTSD, the person must experience a traumatic event[16] and have an emotional reaction to that event. Thus, when studying the epidemiology of PTSD, it is critical to test the prevalence of various traumas within a community, the characteristics of individuals who develop PTSD after a traumatic event and any risk factors of individuals who are likely to be exposed to trauma. Symptoms of PTSD, which can occur anywhere from a few weeks after the traumatic event to years later, include, but are not limited to, numbing, reexperiencing the traumatic event and avoidance of triggers of the trauma.[17] According to McFarlane, trauma can devastate individuals emotionally and physically, and the public health community must be committed to prevent the damage caused by PTSD.[18] As Boehnlein notes in his article "Culture and Society in Posttraumatic Stress Disorder: Implication for Psychotherapy," the symptoms associated with PTSD are fairly uniform and include nightmares, startle reactions, inability to sleep, detachment from others, survivor's guilt, memory problems and avoiding triggers of the traumatic event.[19]

Much of the literature that examines PTSD stressors focuses on catastrophic natural disasters, violent episodes or other cataclysmic events.[20] Storms, droughts and floods are often the episodes associated with inducing PTSD.[21] Under the DSM-IV, besides the previous criteria for a PTSD stressor designated in the DSM-III, the authors added that the trauma must induce "intense fear, helplessness or horror."

According to Friedman, "PTSD is stimulus-driven.…[S]timuli that resemble the trauma will bring that trauma back to the victims. So part of PTSD involves numbing, emotional shutdown and avoidance."[22] The stressor to which an individual is exposed, and whether this stressor qualifies as a PTSD stressor, is a primary concern in evaluating PTSD. In the 1996 Detroit Area Survey of Trauma, the lifetime prevalence of traumatic exposure was 89.6 percent, with the mean number of traumatic situations at 4.8 percent.[23] The belief was that the traumatic exposure level was so elevated because the types of stressors those surveyed reported were broad.[24]

PTSD was formally introduced as a psychological diagnosis in 1980. As mentioned elsewhere in this book, while individuals can suffer the psychological effects of a traumatic event, one hallmark of PTSD is the delayed onset of symptoms, with sufferers exhibiting signs weeks, months or years after the initial event.[25] One debate regarding PTSD in the Civil War is whether Civil War soldiers experienced psychological trauma in the same ways as soldiers of other wars. The evidence and research suggests that, in fact, they did. This is one of the areas this book will seek to inform through memoirs, diaries, research and other primary and secondary sources.[26] One source in particular that seems to point to the Civil War being a PTSD-triggering event has its roots in the manner in which soldiers fought during the war.[27] From firearms to disease and postwar life, the seeds of trauma were ripe to be planted for many who took part in the conflict.[28]

In 2013, the American Psychiatric Association revised the PTSD diagnostic criteria in the fifth edition:

Posttraumatic Stress Disorder (PTSD) will be included in a new chapter in DSM-5 on Trauma- and Stress-or-Related Disorders. This move from DSM-IV, which addressed PTSD as an anxiety disorder, is among several changes approved for this condition that is increasingly at the center of public as well as professional discussion. The diagnostic criteria for the manual's next edition identify the trigger to PTSD as exposure to actual or threatened death, serious injury or sexual violation. The exposure must result from one or more of the following scenarios, in which the individual: directly experiences the traumatic event; witnesses the traumatic event in person; learns that the traumatic event occurred to a close family member or close friend (with the actual or threatened death being either violent or accidental); or experiences first-hand repeated or extreme exposure to aversive details of the traumatic event (not through media, pictures, television or movies unless work-related). The disturbance, regardless of its trigger, causes clinically significant distress or impairment in the individual's social interactions, capacity to work or other important areas of functioning. It is not the physiological result of another medical condition, medication, drugs or alcohol. Changes in PTSD Criteria Compared to DSM-IV, the diagnostic criteria for DSM-5 draw a clearer line when detailing what constitutes a traumatic event. Sexual assault is specifically included, for example, as is a recurring exposure that could apply to police officers or first responders. Language stipulating an individual's response to the event—intense fear, helplessness or horror, according to DSM-IV—has been deleted because that criterion proved to have no utility in predicting the onset of PTSD. DSM-5 pays more attention to the behavioral symptoms that accompany PTSD and proposes four distinct diagnostic clusters instead of three. They are described as re-experiencing, avoidance, negative cognitions and mood, and arousal. Re-experiencing covers spontaneous memories of the traumatic event, recurrent dreams related to it, flashbacks or other intense or prolonged psychological distress. Avoidance refers to distressing memories, thoughts, feelings or external reminders of the event. Negative cognitions and mood represents myriad feelings, from a persistent and distorted sense of blame of self or others, to estrangement from others or markedly diminished interest in activities, to an inability to remember key aspects of the event. Finally, arousal is marked by aggressive, reckless or self-destructive behavior, sleep disturbances, hyper-vigilance or related problems. The current manual emphasizes the "flight" aspect associated with PTSD; the criteria of DSM-5 also account for the "fight" reaction often seen.

Further,

The number of symptoms that must be identified depends on the cluster. DSM-5 would only require that a disturbance continue for more than a month and would eliminate the distinction between acute and chronic phases of PTSD….Certain military leaders, both active and retired, believe the word "disorder" makes many soldiers who are experiencing PTSD symptoms reluctant to ask for help. They have urged a change to rename the disorder posttraumatic stress injury, a description that they say is more in line with the language of troops and would reduce stigma. But others believe it is the military environment that needs to change, not the name of the disorder, so that mental health care is more accessible and soldiers are encouraged to seek it in a timely fashion. Some attendees at the 2012 APA Annual Meeting, where this was discussed in a session, also questioned whether injury is too imprecise a word for a medical diagnosis. In DSM-5, PTSD will continue to be identified as a disorder.[29]

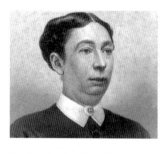

Sophronia Bucklin. *Library of Congress, Washington, D.C.*

PTSD AND RACISM

In thinking through stressors for trauma, an important one for African American soldiers and African American healthcare workers during the Civil War was racism. A key factor also has to do with secondary trauma. African American soldiers entered the war uniquely in terms of racism and trauma, and some horrors experienced during the war would have served as secondary or tertiary traumas. Racism has been defined as "the belief that race accounts for differences in human character or ability and that a particular race is superior to others."[30] The *Dictionary of Cultural Literacy* defines racism as "[t]he belief that some races are inherently superior (physically, intellectually or culturally) to others, and therefore have a right to dominate them. In the United States, racism, particularly by whites against blacks, has created profound racial tension and conflict in virtually all aspects of American society."[31]

According to Scurfield, "Race-related experiences can be defined as experiences that occur solely or primarily because of one's racial status and/

or race-based physical appearance. Such exposure could be considered as a possible environmental stressor in the etiology of the adjustment and stress disorders."[32]

Further, African Americans and other racial minorities can experience racism in life-threatening terms. Scurfield speaks about an African American Vietnam veteran who reported that "while in a latrine four white soldiers began verbally taunting and threatening him. They called him to do anything about it. Outnumbered, he felt threatened for his physical safety, and did not say anything back to the four white soldiers. They laughed and sneered at him and finally let him leave the latrine."[33]

In order to examine epidemiology, racial discrimination and PTSD, a general search of post-traumatic stress disorder revealed thousands of articles; a search of "African Americans" and "post-traumatic stress disorder" revealed thousands of articles as well; a search of "African Americans," "black" and "post-traumatic stress disorder" yielded dozens of articles. There are certain scholarly works that examine PTSD as it relates to ethnicity and specifically African Americans. In a piece titled "Ethnicity and Traumatic Stress: The Intersecting Point in Psychotherapy," Parson asserts that "unless ethnic variables are taken into account, interventions are bound to fail."[34] Valuable sources as to the varying ways blacks react to stress can be found in Vietnam War–era veteran studies.

While involvement in heavy combat was the most crucial factor in severe forms of post-traumatic stress reactions and symptoms for African American Vietnam veterans, being in the war environment produced stress-related symptoms. Approximately 70 percent of African American veterans of heavy combat suffered stress-related symptoms. According to Parson, this high percentage can be accounted for in several ways: first, many African American veterans had a psychological identification with Vietnamese civilians. Second, African Americans as a group have a "stress-primed" orientation to life.[35] This second factor is critical in the study of trauma and African American soldiers during the Civil War.

Allen seems to concur with Parson's "stress-primed orientation" theory. In his article "PTSD among African Americans," he notes, "African Americans have coped with difficult and oppressive life circumstances from 1619 to present times....African Americans have made progress through legal and political and economic action, but for most, the marginality and conditionality of being African American in America remains a fact of everyday life."[36] According to Allen, "benign neglect," institutional racism, poverty and general debasement have severely tested the psyches of African Americans.[37]

Ultimately, there is a solid amount of literature that shows that African American Vietnam veterans have higher rates of PTSD than their white counterparts;[38] that African Americans, while experiencing more severe bouts of PTSD, drop out of treatment sooner than Caucasians; and that African Americans may have a greater susceptibility to PTSD. According to Priscilla Schulz, "[R]esearchers suggest that differences in economic factors between African Americans and Caucasian Americans, and higher levels of exposure to trauma in the lives of African Americans may explain these results."[39]

Herman speaks to the "legacy of slavery" in her work *Trauma and Recovery*. In an insightful passage, she declares:

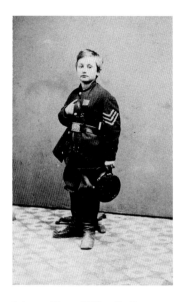

Johnny Clem. *Wikimedia Commons.*

> [T]*he unhealed racial divisions of our country create an ongoing potential for violence. The worst civil disturbance of the past few years, the Los Angeles riots, were provoked by the failure of the justice system to hold armed white police officers accountable for the severe beating of an unarmed black man. Within the African-American community, it was widely understood that such abuses were political crimes, carried out as part of a systematic pattern of racial oppression. The issue at trial was whether the larger society would condone the most flagrant of these human rights abuses. The responsibility to bear witness fell to the jury in the criminal trial. In their refusal to see the crime that was documented before their eyes, we can recognize the familiar defenses of denial, distancing and dissociation. As is so often the case, the bystanders chose to identify with the perpetrators rather than with the victim, and it was this betrayal, not simply the violence of the police, that unleashed a communal outbreak of murderous rage.*[40]

According to Herman, "Racism and historical oppression have created barriers of mistrust for young men of color."[41]

As Allen and others have pointed out, the breadth of research specific to African Americans and PTSD is far from extensive: "There is a paucity of accurate epidemiological data on the incidence and distribution of PTSD."[42] The studies that do exist seem to fairly conclusively point to the link between being African American and an increased likelihood of developing PTSD.[43]

According to Dr. Matthew Friedman for the National Center for PTSD,

> *Soldiers' heart or irritable heart was marked by a rapid pulse, anxiety, and trouble breathing. US Doctor Jacob Mendes Da Costa studied Civil War Soldiers with these cardiac symptoms and described it as overstimulation of the heart's nervous system or Da Costa's syndrome. Soldiers were often returned to battle after receiving drugs to control symptoms. In 1952, the American Psychiatric Association (APA) produced the first Diagnostic and Statistical Manual of Mental Disorders (DSM-I), which included "gross stress reaction."*[44]

The diagnosis was proposed for people who had symptoms from traumatic events such as disaster or combat. A problem was that this diagnosis assumed that reactions to trauma would resolve themselves relatively quickly; if symptoms were still present after six months, another diagnosis had to be made. Despite growing evidence that trauma exposure was associated with psychiatric problems, this diagnosis was eliminated in the second edition of DSM (1968). DSM-II included "adjustment reaction to adult life," which was clearly insufficient to characterize a PTSD-like condition.

The diagnosis was limited to three examples of trauma: unwanted pregnancy with suicidal thoughts, fear linked to military combat and the Ganser syndrome (marked by incorrect answers to questions) in prisoners facing a death sentence. In 1980, APA added PTSD to DSM-III, which stemmed from research involving returning Vietnam War veterans, Holocaust survivors, sexual trauma victims and others. Links between the trauma of war and post-military civilian life was established. The DSM-III criteria for PTSD were revised in DSM-III-R (1987), DSM-IV (1994), DSM-IV-TR (2000) and DSM-5 (2013) to reflect continuing research. One important finding that was not clear at first is that PTSD is relatively common. Recent data shows about four out of every one hundred American men (4 percent) and ten out of every one hundred American women (10 percent) will be diagnosed with PTSD in their lifetimes. An important change in DSM-5 is that PTSD is no longer classified as an anxiety disorder. PTSD is sometimes associated with other mood states (for example, depression) and with angry or reckless behavior rather than anxiety. PTSD includes four different types of symptoms: relieving the

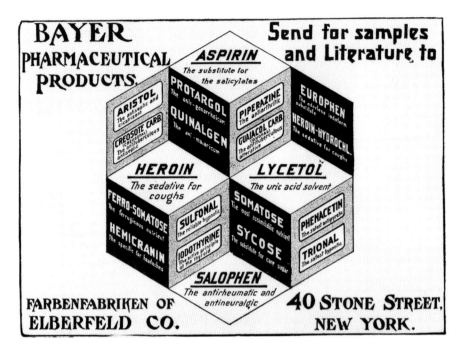

Bayer Pharmaceuticals. *Wikimedia Commons.*

traumatic event (also called reexperience or intrusion), avoiding situations that are reminders of the event, negative changes in beliefs and feelings and hyperarousal or overreactive to situations. Most people experience some of these symptoms after a traumatic event, so PTSD is not diagnosed unless all four types of symptoms last for at least a month and cause significant distress or problems with day-to-day functioning.

EPIDEMIOLOGY OF PTSD

Among some of the most exhaustive studies of the epidemiology of PTSD are those related to Vietnam veterans. While the focus of this book is the Civil War, trauma statistics on Vietnam veterans are instructive and helpful. The National Vietnam Veterans Readjustment Study (NVVRS) was an extensive study on PTSD and Vietnam veterans. Conducted from 1986 to 1988, the NVVRS included interviews with 3,016 American veterans.[45] Among the findings were:

- 30.9 percent of all male Vietnam "theater" veterans have had full-blown PTSD.
- Another 22.5 percent have had partial PTSD.
- Almost 50.0 percent of male Vietnam veterans currently suffering from PTSD have been arrested or arrested at least once.
- 34.2 percent of veterans arrested have been arrested more than once, and 11.5 percent have been convicted of a felony.
- The estimated lifetime prevalence of alcohol abuse or dependence among male veterans is 38.2 percent versus 11.2 percent for the general population.[46]
- 40 percent of Vietnam veterans had been divorced at least once, 10 percent had two or more divorces, 14.1 percent reported high levels of marital problems and 23.1 reported high levels of parenting problems.[47]

An examination of specific stressors shows that civilians exposed to physical attacks have a PTSD prevalence rate of 3.5 percent. Vietnam veterans exposed to physical attacks had a prevalence rate of 6.3 percent.

As mentioned earlier, the Detroit HMO study, with a random sample size of 1,007 individuals, found a lifetime exposure to traumatic events of 39 percent with a rate of PTSD of 23.6 percent and an overall lifetime prevalence rate of 9.2 percent.[48]

One of the largest and most exhaustive studies conducted on the condition was the National Comorbidity Study, which had 8,098 participants. The study, conducted between September 1990 and February 1992, discovered a lifetime PTSD prevalence of 7.8.[49] (60.7 percent of men and 51.2 percent of women reported at least "one traumatic event" such as "being involved in a fire or flood, wartime involvement, [or] being involved in a life-threatening accident."[50])

According to the report, PTSD can be a lifelong illness, with those afflicted being exposed to several traumatic events during their lives.[51]

LEGAL IMPLICATIONS

One of the most fruitful areas for obtaining information about PTSD patterns is in the legal field. While plaintiffs' reactions and responses can be influenced by litigation, lawsuits are one of the first places to which one can turn to find the exploration of the link between traumatic incidents and PTSD.

In PTSD cases, a plaintiff claims that because of the defendant's wrongful actions, the plaintiff has been psychologically injured. As an expert witness, the questions a psychiatrist or a mental health professional has to answer are myriad: Has the plaintiff suffered a psychic injury? Is the injury related to the defendant's actions? What damages should the plaintiff recover?[52]

STRESSORS

In the past, there has been debate regarding the need for a traumatic experience residing "outside the range of usual human experience"[53] in order to induce PTSD.[54] In fact, for many individuals, exposure to trauma is quite frequent.[55] While the DSM has indicated traumas causing PTSD should be outside the range of ordinary trauma, as stated elsewhere in this book, the vast majority of traumas that cause PTSD are "quite common."[56] The list of twelve traumatic events[57] presented to National Comorbidity Survey respondents with the question "did any of these events ever happen to you" included 1. a life-threatening accident, 2. witnessing someone badly injured or killed, 3. rape, 4. sexual molestation, 5. serious physical attack, 6. physical abuse as a child and 7. neglect as a child—all devastating, but not uncommon events.[58]

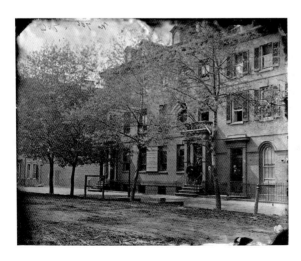

Central Office of Sanitary Commission.
Wikimedia Commons.

CHILDREN AND PTSD

Children are a population crucial to study with respect to PTSD and the Civil War. From soldiers to orphans, sons to daughters, young people played a vital role in pre– and post–Civil War America. According to the research, exposure to violence in young children has a dramatic outcome on future mental health wellness.[59] Adolescents often display reexperiencing symptoms and an inability to develop self-sufficiency, whereas young children are prone to exhibit avoidance tendencies.[60] More common stressors may have a wide range of effects on different individuals, and victimization statistics challenge the assertion that traumatic events are unusual experiences.[61] Compared with major life events, daily stressors have been reported to play a more central role in the development and maintenance of psychological problems.[62] The prevalence and severity of chronic and everyday stressors in the lives of adolescents may predispose them to symptoms of psychological distress.[63] According to Breslau et al., childhood experiences can lead to a variety of mental health issues later in life, including depression, post-traumatic stress disorder and anxiety disorders.[64] Bromet states that traumatic events

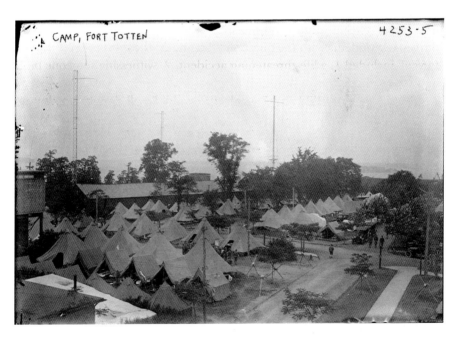

Fort at Willets Point/Fort Totten, Queens, New York. *U.S. National Archives and Records Administration.*

during childhood can lead to antisocial personality disorder, depression, teen pregnancy, drug use and PTSD.[65] Thus, children and adolescents who experience a great deal of trauma, abuse and psychic stress appear to enter adulthood with the ingredients necessary to create PTSD.

IMPLICATIONS FOR THE CIVIL WAR

I used to believe that significant trauma was rare, and that the human psyche, once damaged, was often irreparable.…But I learned two seemingly incongruous truths about us a human beings—that shattering events are more common than we admit, and that, with help, people are incredibly resilient physically, emotionally and spiritually.[66]
—Noah Wyle, actor/entertainer

According to the surgeon general's report "Mental Health: Culture, Race and Ethnicity," "Cultural and social factors have the most direct role in the causation of post-traumatic stress disorder—PTSD."[67] The report concludes that "exposure to trauma is related to the development of subsequent mental disorders in general and of post-traumatic stress disorder (PTSD) in particular."[68]

Much more research needs to be conducted to explore the toll a lifetime of PTSD has on an individual and the implications for those who lived through the horrors of the Civil War. From racism, to combat, to generational trauma, there remains much to be learned. Researchers must continue to embrace the concept that various stressors may lead to PTSD. Research funds should be earmarked for in-depth analysis of this hypothesis. According to Butts, "It is not surprising that, given this disregard of African Americans, responses to racial discrimination by African Americans are often not viewed as severe enough to indicate that these blacks may have post-traumatic stress disorder (PTSD)."[69] PTSD research has shifted from the hypothesis that only the most horrific, uncommon events can provoke PTSD to the understanding that common, though traumatic, events such as rape, robbery, assault and natural disasters are the most prevalent catalysts for the condition.[70] As Kessler et. al. assert, "Despite a growing body of work on the extent to which PTSD is associated with specific traumas, limited epidemiologic data are available that describe the population prevalence of PTSD, the kinds of traumas most strongly associated with PTSD, the demographic correlates of PTSD, the comorbidity of PTSD with other disorders and the typical course of PTSD."[71] Once more studies are done, the next step will be to examine variances within the population.

A great deal of research has been conducted on the offspring of Holocaust victims and the intergenerational transmission of trauma. Novae, in referring to a 1998 study by Yehuda et al., concludes that "offspring of Holocaust survivor parents with PTSD have a higher lifetime risk for PTSD and report more distress after traumatic events." Novae goes on to elaborate: "[B]esides the exposure to their parents' traumatic stories and their trauma-related acquired behavioral patterns, these offspring may have a biological vulnerability to traumatic stress and PTSD transmitted to them from their parents."[72] In studies and interviews of African Americans regarding PTSD and discrimination symptoms, more research is needed on the intergenerational impact of slavery, the Civil War, Reconstruction, segregation and the civil rights movement.[73]

Regarding African Americans, cultural awareness and competency by clinicians and investigators need to be raised. Parson notes that "it may be difficult to determine the degree of psychological impairment with traumatized black clients, because of their culturally determined trained capacity for interior-exterior incongruity."[74] Additionally, "what may be a healthy cultural suspiciousness and adaptive response to the experience of racism may be misdiagnosed as paranoia, with the manifestation of cultural hypervigilance toward non-minority clinicians."[75] As McFarlane points out, "Traumatic events cause demonstrable and chronic long-term effects on psychological and physical health. Attempting to prevent these adverse effects is a critical public health issue. The avoidance of traumatic memories and the ambivalence of victims towards acknowledging their state of mind are major barriers in establishing systems of care and can lead to underestimating the consequences of these events."[76]

The surgeon general's report on mental health, culture, race and ethnicity, under a section titled "Mistrust," affirms that mistrust is a "major barrier" to ensuring that minorities receive the mental health care they need. Further, "mistrust of clinicians by minorities arises, in the broadest sense, from historical persecution and from present-day struggles with racism and discrimination."[77] Like Parson and Butts, Allen also speaks to cultural sensitivity when dealing with PTSD in African Americans. He cites Grier's and Cobbs's (1968) and Carter's (1974) discussions of African Americans wearing the black mask to protect themselves and asserts, "The white therapist must be aware that either an extremely blunted or hyperactive appearance may say as much about the Black client's interactions with the clinician as about the clinicians' basic diagnosis."[78] Butts elaborates: "The tendency on the part of some European Americans to define casually the reality of African-Americans' experience may be problematic in view of the lack of knowledge about the 'black experience' displayed by so many European Americans."

PTSD is devastating and permeates the lives of those afflicted. Studies have shown that individuals with PTSD are six times more likely than controls of similar demographics to attempt suicide.[79] PTSD directly impacts the work, marriage and education of its sufferers.[80] PTSD can also have devastating physical consequences. According to Yehuda, "Exposure to a traumatic event can often explain the presence of nonspecific symptoms such as palpitations, shortness of breath, tremor, nausea, insomnia, unexplained pain, and mood swings, as well as a reluctance to undergo certain types of examinations."[81] Yet according to the U.S. National Comorbidity Survey, among the reasons given by individuals in the survey with PTSD who were not in treatment, 66.2 percent of the men and 60.0 percent of the females felt they "did not have a problem requiring treatment." Of those individuals who felt that they had a problem but did not seek treatment, reasons given included "unsure about where to go [40 percent for men, 49.4 percent for women], treatment was too expensive [46.5 percent men, 48.2 percent women], fear of forced hospitalization [34.6 percent men, 22.0 percent women], and stigma [23.0 percent and 17.3 percent]."[82]

If detected early, PTSD is treatable—with the right intervention. If a segment of our community is suffering from this disease, we as a population must be committed to researching the cause and effect, understanding exacerbating factors and educating individuals on treatment and financing cures.

Physicians, Healthcare Workers and Psychological Trauma in New York and D.C. during and after the War

T he story of Dr. Susan McKinney Steward is one that is exemplary in terms of the trajectory of a post–Civil War African American physician. Her accomplishments include membership in the Kings County and New York State Homeopathic Medical Societies, presenting a paper titled "Colored Women in America" to the 1911 First Universal Races Congress at the University of London, participating in the Women in Medicine National Association of Colored Women's Club Convention and caring for sick servicemen and Buffalo Soldiers in Montana and Wyoming.

Steward's story is a critical one in understanding healthcare in the United States generally and New York specifically after the Civil War.

Susan Maria Smith was born in Brooklyn, New York, in 1847. Her parents were successful farmers, and they were among the elite of Brooklyn's African American community. As a child, Steward learned to play the organ, and she performed as an organist for Siloam Presbyterian Church and the Bridge Street African Methodist Church for many years. Her early education qualified her for teaching positions, and she taught school in Washington, D.C., and New York City. Sylvanus Smith, Steward's father, was a free black man from Brooklyn who was a business owner and property developer in a free black community named Weeksville in honor of James Weeks of Virginia. Smith and others, such as James and Elizabeth Gloucester, William Wilson and James Pennington, settled in Weeksville because by owning land there, they could meet the $250 property requirement for voting that the New York legislature created for black males.[83] Only five years after the

Thirteenth Amendment to the Constitution abolished slavery in the United States, Susan McKinney Steward graduated from medical school and became the first African American woman physician in New York and only the third African American female doctor in the country.[84]

Medicine was a unique career choice for any woman in the mid-nineteenth century, especially for an African American woman. Because women were not welcome in existing male medical schools, all-female institutions opened. In 1867, Steward enrolled in the New York Medical College for Women in Manhattan, where she was living with one of her sisters. [85]

Dr. Clemence Sophia Lozier became Steward's mentor, and the two remained close friends until Lozier's death in 1888. Students at the New York Medical College for Women were required to study anatomy, physiology, chemistry, surgery, obstetrics and medical jurisprudence. Clinical lectures were given at the New York Homeopathic Dispensary. When a lack of funds forced the college to send students to Bellevue Hospital for clinical work, male students frequently bullied female classmates. Although her prosperous parents could have afforded to pay for her medical school education, Steward paid her own tuition with money she earned teaching music in a school in Washington, D.C., for two years.

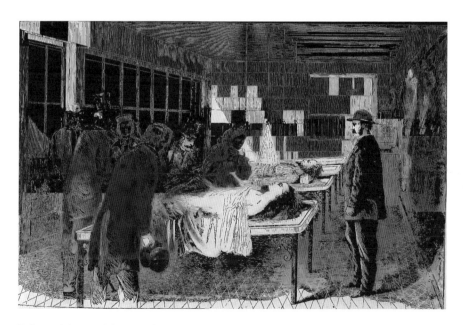

Bellevue Morgue. *Wikimedia Commons.*

Dr. Clemence S. Lozier, Steward's mentor, was born on December 11, 1813, in Plainfield, New Jersey. In 1849, she was admitted to the Central New York College of Rochester and then to the Eclectic College. She graduated in 1853. After practicing medicine for a few years, she decided to start a medical college for women. On November 1, 1873, the New York Medical College opened its doors with seven students and eight faculty members (four men and four women). The school moved from 724 Broadway to Second Avenue and Twelfth Street in June 1868. The school grew over time in stature and reputation. According to her son Dr. A.W. Lozier, "Perhaps no woman of her age has accomplished so much in so many different directions for women. No one ever inspired women more with faith in themselves, nor ever a readier hand worked with a readier heart for mankind." According to her granddaughter Jessica Lozier Payne, "I was eighteen years old when my grandmother, Dr. Clemence S. Lozier, died. My strongest recollection of her is her gracious personality and gentle beauty, with soft curls framing her face. Although forceful in character, she gained results by persuasion and example. Many and difficult were her problems, but sustained and inspired by her active faith, she solved them, and won a prominent place in the medical profession, consulting with Dr. Jacoby, Dr. Janeway and Dr. Helmuth. She was a warm friend of Susan B. Anthony and Elizabeth Cady Stanton."[86]

When Steward graduated from medical school at the top of her class in 1870, she established a medical practice in her Brooklyn home, which she ran from 1870 to 1895. Her patients made up a diverse group and affectionately called her Dr. Susan. Some had been directly touched by the events of the Civil War. Dr. Steward became widely known, and she opened another office in Manhattan. She achieved wealth and a local reputation as a successful physician with an interracial clientele. Dr. Steward excelled, especially in prenatal and pediatric care, which became her specialty. She maintained her offices in Brooklyn and Manhattan for many years and treated a variety of patients regardless of income or ethnicity.[87]

In 1871, Susan married William G. McKinney, an Episcopal minister from South Carolina who was seventeen years her senior. The couple lived in Steward's parents' home until 1874, when they moved to a predominantly white area of Brooklyn. The couple had two children: Anna, who became a schoolteacher, and William Sylvanus, who became an Episcopal priest.

In 1890, William McKinney suffered a cerebral hemorrhage and could not work. Susan supported the family, in addition to six of her relatives, who lived in her home. William McKinney died in 1892. Steward was active

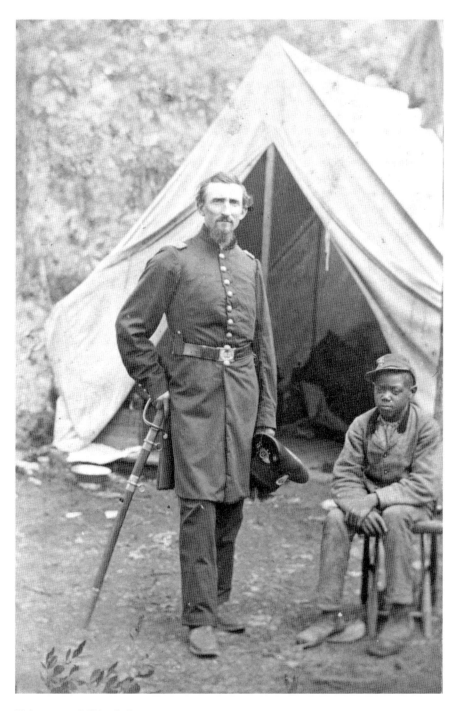

Union camp. *Wikimedia Commons*.

in the Kings County Homeopathic Medical Society and Homeopathic Medical Society of the State of New York. In the 1880s, she presented two important papers to the New York group—the first about a pregnant woman who was incorrectly treated, the second about childhood diseases. She was a founding member of the Alumni Association of the New York Medical College for Women and taught at the school in 1882–83. During the 1880s and early 1890s, in addition to her medical practice, Dr. Steward was active in establishing medical facilities for African

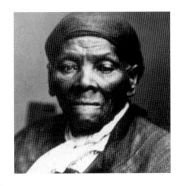

Harriet Tubman. *Library of Congress, Washington, D.C.*

Americans and the aged. She was one of the founders of the Brooklyn Women's Homeopathic Hospital and Dispensary (1881), which served the African American community, and she worked as a surgeon on the staff. During these years, Dr. Steward also continued her medical education; she was the only woman in a postgraduate class at Long Island College Hospital in Brooklyn (1887–88).

Besides surgical rounds at the Brooklyn Women's Homeopathic Hospital and Dispensary, Dr. Steward was a physician for the elderly at the Brooklyn Home for Aged Colored People, where she also served as a board member (1892–95). She also found time in her busy schedule to practice at New York Medical College and Hospital for Women in Manhattan (1892–96). Taking part in social reform issues of the day, Dr. Steward became a member of the Women's Local Union of New York (a leading black women's club) and the Equal Suffrage League of Brooklyn. She was active in Bridge Street's missionary work and was president of the Woman's Christian Temperance Union Number 6. At the Brooklyn Literary Union, she organized musical programs and sold tickets to musical events. Steward maintained a love of music throughout her life. As a child, she took lessons from famed organists John Zundel and Henry Eyre Brown. In her youth, she had served as the organist and choir director for the Siloam Presbyterian and Bridge Street AME Churches. She also contributed to many of the Brooklyn Literary Union's musical programs, often accompanied by her children, who shared her talent.

Susan married Theophilus Gould Steward on November 26, 1896; he was an ordained minister and chaplain of the Twenty-Fifth U.S. Colored Infantry. They were known as the Buffalo Soldiers, the name given to them by the Native American tribes they were fighting. Congress established this unit as the first peacetime all-black regiment in the regular U.S. Army. After having spent her entire life in Brooklyn, Dr. Steward moved several times, as Reverend Steward was stationed at various army posts in the West. She earned multiple medical licenses and practiced medicine in Montana and Wyoming. After the Civil War, the army expanded to forty-five infantry regiments, and four regiments of African American soldiers were created, the Thirty-Eighth, Thirty-Ninth, Fortieth and Forty-First Infantries. On March 3, 1869, the four regiments were consolidated into one under the command of Colonel Joseph A. Mower. The Stewards also traveled. From 1898 to 1902, Reverend Steward was working in Cuba and the Philippines. In 1898, Wilberforce University in Ohio hired Dr. Steward as a resident physician and a health and nutrition teacher. In 1902, the reverend was stationed at Fort Niobrara, Nebraska, and Susan joined him there. In 1906, the Stewards moved to Fort McIntosh, near Laredo, Texas. After leaving Texas, Dr. Steward returned to her job at Wilberforce University, and Reverend Steward joined the faculty as a history teacher.

In 1911, the Stewards attended the First Universal Races Congress in London. The meeting brought together Africans, Asians, Americans and Europeans seeking to improve relationships and cooperation between the East and West. Dr. Steward, an accomplished public speaker, presented a paper at the conference titled "Colored American Women," which dealt with achievements of famous African American women, including Phyllis Wheatley, Ida Wells Barnett and Mary Church Terrell. In 1914, Dr. Steward delivered a speech, "Women in Medicine," before the National Association of Colored Women's Clubs in Wilberforce, Ohio. In this lecture, she examines the history of women in medicine from biblical times to 1914. Steward concluded that there was no need for separate medical schools for women and they should have equal opportunity for internships. Furthermore:

> *Fortunate are the men who marry these women* [doctors] *from an economic standpoint....They are blessed in a three-fold measure...* [taking] *unto themselves a wife, a trained nurse, and a doctor....*[I caution such women] *to avoid becoming unevenly yoked...such a companion will prove to be a millstone hanged around her neck.*

Dr. Susan McKinney Steward died suddenly on March 7, 1918, at Wilberforce University. Her body was returned to Brooklyn for burial in Green-Wood Cemetery. At her funeral, Hallie Quinn Brown delivered the eulogy. Dr. William S. Scarborough, president of Wilberforce University, and author Dr. W.E.B. DuBois also spoke at the funeral.

Hallie Quinn Brown's eulogy included this description of Steward:

> *She was great in the estimation of those who knew her capacity, her ability, her real worth….She was modest. A woman absolutely self-reliant, honest to herself and to her friends. She was one of those generous natures that love peace, order, and harmony. But she could strike, and strike hard, in what she believed to be a righteous cause. With her it was justice on the one side, and injustice on the other.*

In 1974, the New York Board of Education named a Brooklyn school in her honor: Dr. Susan Smith McKinney Junior High School. In the 1980s, African American women doctors in New York, New Jersey and Connecticut named their medical society after McKinney.[88] McKinney was an activist in her own right, and this had positive effects on the post–Civil War generation. An example is an art exhibit she had in her home at 205 DeKalb Avenue to raise funds for the 1893 Women's Loyal Union to combat lynchings. Dr. Steward was an important medical figure in the post–Civil War era, and while her practice focus was children, she also cared for soldiers and the physical and psychological pain they suffered.[89]

Dr. Susan McKinney Steward's story is compelling because of the barriers she broke, the obstacles she overcame and the patients she cared for. She cared for patients affected both directly and indirectly by the Civil War. Her personal and medical trajectory are enlightening from a pre– and post–Civil War perspective. In particular, for the purposes of this book, the care to those postwar who were on the road to recovery and the roadblocks they encountered while under Steward's care is instructive.

NOSTALGIA

Another word closely linked with psychological trauma was *nostalgia*. Nostalgia was closely related to homesickness. Homesickness that seemed to linger or worsen was often called nostalgia. The numbers of reported nostalgia cases were in the thousands, but it is clear it was probably an underreported disease, especially as it related to soldiers discharged because of nostalgia.[90]

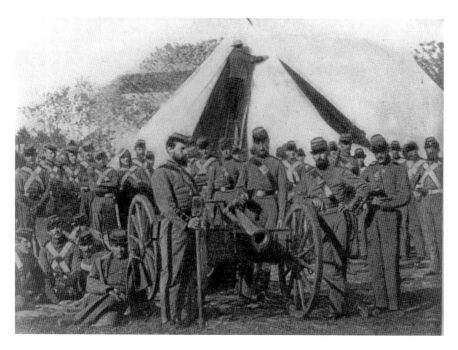

Seventh New York Militia. *Library of Congress, Washington, D.C.*

An oft-repeated concept in this book is that there was no recognized diagnosis of PTSD during the Civil War, and thus, various phrases were used to describe it. *Homesickness* was one such term. According to the U.S. Sanitary Commission (USSC), homesickness was very difficult for physicians to treat. Medicine was ineffective, but the cases were real.

Symptoms of nostalgia included weeping, groaning, longing for home, desire for solitude, hallucinations, loss of appetite, cardiac pain and a vacant gaze.[91] Treatment during the war varied wildly, from trying to reason with soldiers to helping the soldier "laugh" his way out of his mood and regain a sense of camaraderie with fellow soldiers. Conversely, other physicians believed sympathy and compassion were the way to deal with soldiers suffering from nostalgia.

The role of the Women's Central Association of Relief (WCAR) was to coordinate relief efforts, coordinate with the army's medical department on needs and train nurses. There was also a fair amount of interface with civilians. Because of concerns and partnering with civilian organizations, the U.S. Sanitary Commission was born. The WCAR remained a separate entity, serving as an auxiliary to the USSC, supplying not only physical

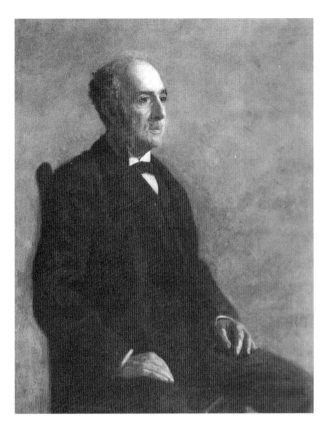

Left: Jacob Mendes Da Costa. *Library of Congress, Washington, D.C.*

Below: The steamer *Lizzie Baker*. *Wikimedia Commons.*

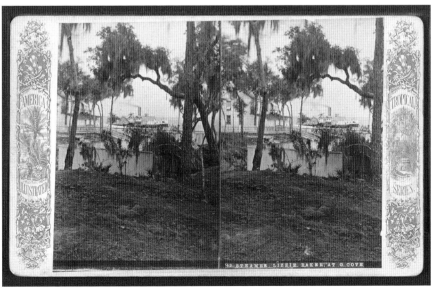

supplies but also emotional support through its network. In their second report, the WCAR administrators stated that "[i]t gives us pleasure to mention that our auxiliaries have shown an increasing willingness to make their contributions correspond to the demand; so that although the total amount of receipts has diminished greatly, the character of the donations has improved so much that we have been enabled to furnish our full proportion of the most valuable articles required, such as woolen shirts, drawers, and socks."[92] In 1862, Charles Brace Loring wrote to F.L. Olmsted, the head of the Sanitary Commission, to ascertain whether he could help in the wartime effort. Olmstead replied with the following letter:

> *Dear Charley: I employ three classes, surgeons, nurses and women—the first and last of two grades, but in neither of either would you yoke. For nurses, I find that any not very sick common soldiers, Yankee, Irish or German, are better than any volunteers. Don't want them. Consequently, don't want you. I have seen enough of it, and it is not an entertainment to which I would invite a friend.*[93]

Another woman who was critical in supporting soldiers was Elizabeth Blackwell. Elizabeth Blackwell was born on February 3, 1821, in Bristol, England. Her family moved to New York City in 1832 and Cincinnati in 1838. Later, Blackwell became a teacher, first in Kentucky and later in North Carolina. She prepared for medical studies, with the hope of being admitted into a school in Philadelphia.

In October 1847, Blackwell was accepted as a medical student at Hobart and William Smith Colleges (Geneva Medical College) in upstate New York and on January 23, 1849, she was the first woman to receive a medical degree in the United States. Blackwell returned to Europe to pursue additional training; she sadly contracted ophthalmia neonatorum, an eye infection, and had to have her left eye removed. She returned to New York City and started her practice at the New York Infirmary for Indigent Women and Children.

When the Civil War began, one of the many logistical issues involved how to get supplies distributed. Mary Ashton Livermore, USSC manager, described early efforts to get supplies to soldiers as a disaster. Between fermenting meat, useless velvet slippers and decaying fruit, something needed to be done. Blackwell organized four thousand women and created the Women's Central Association Relief in New York City. It expanded nationally, distributing bandages, food, clothes and much more. Supplies were critical to the physical and mental well-being of soldiers.

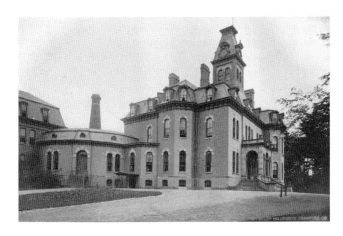

Willard State Hospital.
Library of Congress,
Washington, D.C.

Certain companies helped facilitate this effort. According to the Sanitary Commission's Accounting within the report,

> *To enable our auxiliaries to expand all the money they may be able to collect*
> *for materials, the prices of which have increased so much, our Association*
> *will, for the present, pay all transportation charges on sanitary supplies*
> *delivered at No. 10 Cooper Union. We would, at the same time, remind*
> *our friends that the American Express Company brings all boxes sent by*
> *them free of charge. This has been their uniform practice and has proved*
> *a most valuable donation in aid of the cause. The United States and the*
> *National Express Companies, as also the Harlem, New Haven and Long*
> *Island Railroads, have promised, through their presidents, "to transport all*
> *packages free of charge from places along their lines for the United States*
> *Sanitary Commission."*[94]

As discussed throughout the book, the psychological and the physical often collide to make a strict psychological diagnosis impossible. As many modern-day psychiatrists and psychologists assert, the mind and the body truly are intertwined. Some Civil War surgeons noted heart-related symptoms in patients early in the war. In 1862, surgeon A.J. McKelway reported heart disease caused by "overexertion preceding the battle and excitement and effort during its continuance." With the benefit of two decades of hindsight, the surgeon general's history observed:

> *Overaction of the heart during an engagement was due perhaps as much*
> *to nervous excitement and anticipation of danger as to overexertion. Even*
> *soldiers accustomed to the alarms of battle were not at all times exempt from*

the results of mental impressions. Many cases arrived in hospitals after the continued exertion, anxieties, and excitement. Some patients experienced acute chest pain even while asleep.[95]

Famed author and Civil War nurse Louisa May Alcott, writing about a particular patient she treated from New Jersey, noted that "his mind had suffered more than his body." She described his demeanor and actions: "He lay cheering his comrades on, hurrying them back, then counting them as they fell around him, often clutching my arm, to drag me from the vicinity of a bursting shell, or covering up his head to screen himself from a shower of shot; while an incessant stream of defiant shouts, whispered warnings, and broken laments poured from his lips."[96]

In 1862, acting assistant surgeon Jacob M. Da Costa reported a disease called "Chickahominy fever" among soldiers returning from Major General George B. McClellan's Peninsula Campaign. "Both body and mind remain for a considerable period enfeebled," noted Da Costa. Symptoms included memory loss and "mental wandering." Another surgeon listed such symptoms as "indifferentism, wandering and muttering, restlessness, insomnia, and watchfulness."[97]

Da Costa described typical cases with heart-related symptoms, including "palpitation and a feeling of uneasiness in the cardiac region." Another patient had palpitations and sharp chest pains. The patient's other symptoms improved, and he regained his strength, "but any excitement or labor agitates him and brings on violent beating of the heart," Da Costa observed. "The irritable state of the organ remaining long after the general health was in every other respect fully reestablished, all form a clinical combination of very great interest and frequency."[98] Later,

Da Costa used the phrase "irritable heart" in the title of an 1871 journal article in which he summed up his experience with more than 300 soldiers and continued to define it as a functional cardiac disorder. Besides palpitations, sometimes violent, Da Costa noted that his patients suffered from "smothering or suffocating sensations at night, a mere feeling of uneasiness near the heart, shortness of breath, giddiness, and disturbed sleep, including dreams of unpleasant character."[99]

Da Costa believed approximately 38.5 percent of the cases could be attributed to hard field service, particularly excessive marching. Within this category, he included heavy duty on the picket line, active movements in

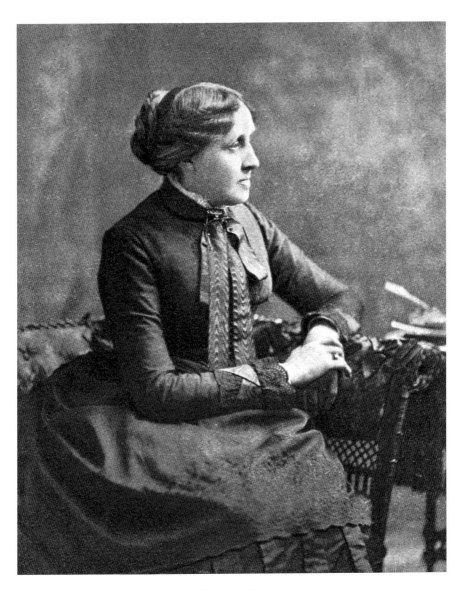

Louisa May Alcott. *Library of Congress, Washington, D.C.*

the face of an enemy, forced marches and arduous and exciting fighting and marching. It differed quite dramatically from other physicians' assessments of battle-related activities during the war. In contrast to an overall lack of treatment for mental disease, there were some treatments in place for heart disease. Da Costa first prescribed rest but also employed plant-based remedies, including digitalis, aconite, veratrum viride, gelsemium, hyoscyamus (henbane), belladonna and atropine, conium (hemlock) and Cannabis indica.[100] By the late nineteenth century, many healthcare workers treating veterans referred to this confluence of symptoms as simply "the war."[101]

Some difficulty in diagnosing trauma and treating postwar effects lies in war's magnitude.[102] However, as the war progressed, it became evident that soldiers, as well as noncombatants such as doctors and nurses, were suffering non-physical ailments because of their wartime experiences.[103] This work's focus on opium and morphine is due in no small measure to the fact that healthcare providers during and after the war attempted to treat many of the symptoms we suspect were related to wartime trauma with these drugs. This appears to have led, sometimes, to what resembles modern-day addiction.[104]

Georgeanna Wolsey, a nurse during the war, recounts her time treating the wounded. Note the language she uses with respect to her transforming feelings around witnessing pain, injuries and death:

> On stacks of marble slabs, we spread mattresses, and out the sickest men. As the number increased, camp beds were set up between glass cases in the outer room and we alternated—typhoid fever, cog wheels and patent churns, typhoid fever, balloons and mouse traps....Here for weeks, went on a sort of hospital picnic. We scrambled through with what we had to do....Here for weeks we worked among these men, cooking for them, feeding them, washing them, sliding them along on their tables, while we climbed upon something and made us their beds with brooms, putting the same powders down their throats with the same spoon, all up and down what seemed half a mile of uneven floor; waxing back to life some of the most unpromising—watching the youngest and best die.

In May 1862, speaking of tending to a wounded soldier, Wolsey writes: "We are changed by all this contact with terror, else how could I deliberately turn my lantern on his face and say to the Doctor behind me 'Is that man dead' And stand coolly, while he listened and examined and pronounced him dead. I could not have quietly said a year ago 'that will make one more bed, Doctor.'"[105]

The Soldier's Life in New York and D.C. during and after the War

D id soldiers of the American Civil War suffer from post-traumatic stress disorder and other psychological disorders? Based on the evidence in this book, it seems that soldiers of the American Civil War did indeed suffer from post-traumatic stress and other psychological disorders.[106]

This chapter will focus on stories and letters from soldiers and how they relate to postwar trauma.

One conclusion drawn from the Civil War is that trauma does not seem to discriminate, as evidenced by the sad case of Randall S. Mackenzie:

> *Post-traumatic stress disorder in the Civil War was no respecter of rank—common soldiers were by no means the only ones who suffered. Senior Civil War leaders, particularly those who consistently "led from the front" were also victimized by it. One of these praised by Ulysses S. Grant as the Union Army's most promising young officer was Randall S. Mackenzie. Graduating first in his West Point class of 1862, Mackenzie achieved the rank of major general of volunteers through his daring leadership in some of the war's fiercest battles, including Second Bull Run, Antietam, Gettysburg, the Overland Campaign, Petersburg, Cedar Creek and Five Forms. He was wounded in six of these battles [which contributed] not only to his aggressive style of command, but also starkly indicative of the intense combat he endured throughout his Civil War Service. Yet the PTSD symptoms that afflicted Mackenzie (and which, in fact, would*

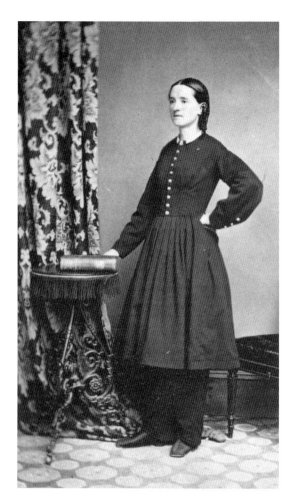

Right: Mary Walker. *Library of Congress, Washington, D.C.*

Below: Twenty-Sixth Regiment, United States Colored Troops. *New York Correction History Society.*

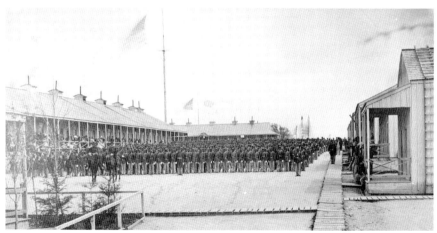

contribute to his death at the age of 48) did not first appear until years after the war.…[B]y 1883, a year after his promotion to Regular Army brigadier general, 12 years of arduous frontier service, closely following his Civil War ordeals, had left Mackenzie physically and emotionally exhausted. One of his subordinates described Mackenzie as continuously "irritable, irascible, exacting…erratic and frequently explosive." In fact, Mackenzie had already suffered a nervous breakdown in 1881, and his seven combat wounds continued to torment him. His behavior became increasingly erratic—extreme emotions, highs and lows, unprovoked violent outbursts, estrangement from others, feelings of persecution. Despite some lucid periods, Mackenzie's obviously severe PTSD symptoms forced his superiors into action. In December 1883, Mackenzie was escorted to the Bloomingdale Asylum for the Insane in New York City and diagnosed with "paralysis of the insane" (a neuropsychiatric disorder also known as paralytic dementia). On March 24, 1884 he was medically retired from the Army, and in June was released to his relatives' care. Mackenzie died at his sister's home on Staten Island, N.Y., on January 19, 1889.[107]

By analyzing the records of hospitals and institutions, it is evident that some Civil War soldiers suffered from PTSD and that the health crisis of the war was more profound than previously thought. Still, several challenges remain as historians try to realign the history of the Civil War to account for its psychological consequences. For one, privacy laws in some states make it difficult for historians to access the Civil War–era medical records needed to pursue further research on PTSD.

Nineteenth-century soldiers, their relatives and physicians also lacked a single descriptor for the symptoms of PTSD. As a result, researchers must decipher outdated language in hospital and pension records, letters and memoirs.

Lastly, as modern-day controversies over veterans' healthcare remind us, mental healthcare providers still struggle to detect and effectively treat PTSD in combat veterans. As a better clinical definition of PTSD emerges, historians continue to reevaluate areas of the Civil War that were once thought to be settled in the history books.[108]

Traumatic brain injury, while familiar in modern days, was not a diagnosis during or after the Civil War. Yet some of the symptoms, including amnesia, excessive sleep and personality changes, may have overlapped with a trauma diagnosis.[109] Some historians and mental health providers have come to believe that combatants during the Civil War suffered from these diseases as well.[110] Diseases such as generalized anxiety disorder and depression may also have afflicted soldiers during the war.

An important article that helps give us some insight regarding trauma and the Civil War is "Physical and Mental Health Costs of Traumatic War Experiences among Civil War Veterans," by Judith Pizarro. The objective of the article was to "identify the role of trauma in war experiences in predicting post-war nervous and physical disease and mortality using archival data from military and medical records of veterans from the Civil War."[111] Pizarro states that "war is particularly traumatic for soldiers because it often involves intimate violence, including witnessing death through direct combat, viewing the enemy before or after killing them, and watching friends and comrades die."[112] According to Pizarro, it is critical to identify the exact combat experiences that are causing the trauma in order to ascertain how detrimental it will be for a particular soldier. Pizarro speaks about intimate violence at length, stating that "[d]uring the Civil War, soldiers were particularly vulnerable to intimate violence. Family members and friends were often assigned to the same company of around 100 men, who were not replaced as they died. When companies suffered substantial losses, survivors were left with few remaining friends or male family members."[113] While guns and cannons were used, the Civil War saw a great deal of both frontal assault and hand-to-hand combat. This resulted in very little buffer for soldiers, with exposure to dead bodies, maimed friends and other horrific sights being fairly common. Some factors Pizarro identified as being predictive of worsening of symptoms include age at enlistment, socioeconomic status and trauma history.[114] Pizarro also has some interesting insights into prisoners of war and trauma. Prisoners of war are a powerful population to examine because of the intense psychic stress they endure. Pizzaro concluded that "although physical hardiness may have acted as a buffer for physical disease it did not protect against the ill effects of war on mental health.…[I]ndividuals who experience severe, prolonged stress may engage in compensatory negative health behaviors such as overeating, smoking, drug abuse or other harmful habits that may lead to subsequent physical disease."[115]

This notion of the mental and physical manifesting somatic symptoms is rooted in research. Pizarro speaks to findings regarding trauma and physical symptoms alone versus combined with psychological symptoms. According to Pizarro, while there is a mild to moderate correlation between war trauma and physical symptoms, such as upper gastrointestinal distress or cardiac symptoms, there is a very strong connection between war trauma, physical symptoms as described previously and psychological symptoms. Specifically, Pizarro looks at percentage of company killed:

> *Percentage of company killed is likely a powerful variable because it serves as a proxy for a variety of traumatic stressors such as witnessing death or dismemberment, handling dead bodies, traumatic loss of comrades, one's own imminent death, kicking others, and being helpless to prevent others' deaths. In addition, veterans who were younger at enlistment had a 93 percent increased risk of developing signs of comorbid physical and nervous disease.* [116]

Supporting this is author Sarah Ford, who tells the story of Albert Frank:

> *Albert Frank was a soldier in the Union Army. At the Battle of Bermuda Hundred near Richmond, Frank was off the front line and sitting on top of a trench. He offered a drink from his canteen to a fellow soldier sitting next to him. While the soldier was taking his drink, a shell exploded and decapitated the man, covering Frank with blood and pieces of brain. Frank experienced a complete loss of cognitive functioning being unable to speak, communicate or understand his fellow soldiers. He was later found on the floor shaking and making bomb noises. The only thing he would say was "Frank is killed." He was taken to the Government Hospital for the Insane in Washington D.C and declared mentally insane. Witnessing such an intense trauma had affected Frank greatly. He was re-experiencing and reenacting the event and he associated himself to the trauma in a negative way saying he was the one killed. These are indicators of post-traumatic stress disorder.* [117]

In her essay "Suffering in Silence," Ford concludes that while the issue regarding whether Civil War soldiers experienced psychological trauma remains an open question for some experts, for researchers, the issue is a closed topic:

> *The question can be definitively answered; psychological disorders are present in soldiers of the Civil War as a result of combat and or its attributing factors. Without a shadow of a doubt the Civil War psychologically scarred and damaged its soldiers. Those brave men put their "sacrifices upon the altar of freedom" and endured a fate worse than death by living their lives in silent suffering. The presence of psychological effects and disorders are evident in the soldiers of the American Civil War.* [118]

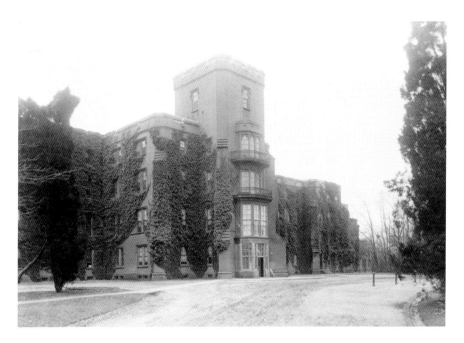

St. Elizabeth's Hospital. *Wikimedia Commons.*

An example of Pizarro's theory of the impact of seeing fellow comrades injured and killed can be found in the Twenty-Sixth Regiment, U.S. Colored Troops (USCT). The Twenty-Sixth was organized at Rikers Island, New York, under the command of Colonel William B. Guernsey.[119] The soldiers spent a good deal of time in South Carolina and were involved in a number of engagements that involved large loss of life. These were recorded in *Dyer's Compendium*, a history of the war's regiments:

> *Reported at Beaufort, S.C., April 13, 1864, and post duty there until November 27. Expedition to Johns and James Islands July 2–10. Operations against Battery Pringle July 4–9. Actions on Johns Island, July 5 and 7. Burden's Causeway July 9. Battle of Honey Hill November 30. Demonstration on Charleston & Savannah Railroad December 6–9. Action at Devaux's Neck December 6. Tillifinny Station December 9. McKay's Point December 22. Ordered to Beaufort, S.C., January 2, 1865, and duty there until August. Mustered out August 28, 1865.*
>
> *Regiment lost during service 2 Officers and 28 Enlisted men killed and mortally wounded and 3 Officers and 112 Enlisted men by disease. Total 145.*

The Twenty-Sixth was involved in some very difficult fights.[120] The expedition to Johns Island and the attempt to take Battery Pringle are good examples. On July 7, 1864, the Twenty-Sixth attacked the Rebel rifle pits with approximately one thousand men. Advancing at first under the cover of woods, the men came upon an open field about two hundred yards from the Rebel line. Charging across, they assaulted the rifle pits frontally and captured them. Then, they pursued fleeing Confederate soldiers, and victory appeared imminent. However, at that point, Rebel reinforcements, the Thirty-Second Georgia Regiment, arrived. The Twenty-Sixth retreated and lost the ground it had already won. The whole engagement on Johns Island was so fierce and produced so many casualties that it became known as "Bloody Bridge," named for the causeway connecting the mainland and the island. Because Confederates often treated black regiments much more harshly when they surrendered or were captured, it must have required an extra measure of courage for an African American to enlist in the U.S. Army for service in the Civil War. Rather than being taken as prisoners, they were often shot in cold blood. When taken as prisoners of war, they could be severely abused. Their white officers suffered as well.

An important individual to help understand the health and well-being of the Twenty-Sixth was hospital steward Noah Elliott. Elliott was born in Kentucky, and on December 24, 1863, he enlisted in Company E of the Twenty-Sixth Infantry, USCT, on Rikers Island, in New York Harbor. On June 30, 1864, he was promoted to hospital steward status and discharged with his unit on August 28, 1865.[121] Elliott was in Lee Township of Athens County in 1865 and 1866, then returned Gallipolis from 1866 to 1874. In 1874, he returned to Lee Township, where he remained until 1884. On August 11, 1886, Dr. Elliott's sister-in-law, Olivia Davidson, married the renowned black educator Booker T. Washington. The house where the marriage took place still stands.

According to his pension record, Dr. Elliott's first wife was Mariah Hughes, who died in Ohio, but in 1915, he called her Maria Pogue. His second wife was Mary A. Davidson, Olivia's sister. They were married in Oswego, New York, in 1862. Mary corresponded with Booker T. Washington on a lifelong basis, even after her sister passed away in 1889. Dr. Elliott died on February 2, 1918, in Columbus, where he had moved after leaving Athens around 1890. According to his obituary in the *Columbus Evening Dispatch*, he was a most devoted physician who "maintained his practice until his illness forced him to give it up about six weeks [prior to his death]." His passing was also noted in the *Journal of the American Medical Association*: "Noah Elliott, Columbus,

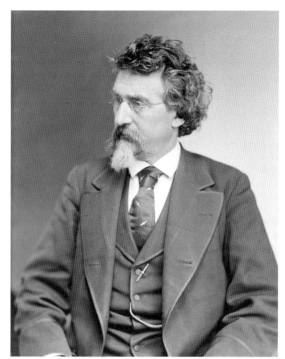

Right: Mathew Brady. *Library of Congress, Washington, D.C.*

Below: Ward University. *Library of Congress, Washington, D.C.*

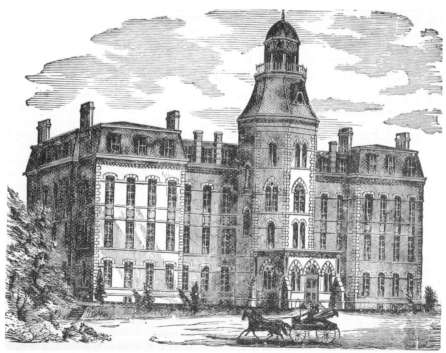

Ohio…aged 92; a colored practitioner; died at his home, February 27, from senile debility [old age]."

David Carll was an African American Cold Spring Harbor resident who fought with the Twenty-Sixth Regiment. Stories like his, a valiant soldier's struggle for compensation, show triumph of healing in the face of trauma.[122] Pension records can be an interesting source of the struggle soldiers endured both to receive payment and to cope with the trauma of war. Struggles such as these can lead to reexperiencing traumatic events. His family found a picture of Carll, thought to be lost, and submitted it to the Bureau of Pensions in 1902. "As part of the final presentation at the African American Civil War Museum, a complete photo copy restoration of the civil war soldier David Carll was revealed and archived for the first time."[123]

With respect to postwar disease, "relative to the oldest enlisted, the [younger soldiers were] more likely to be diagnosed with signs of cardiovascular disease alone and in combination with signs of GI disease and were at greater risk of presenting with signs of comorbid physical and nervous disease."[124] Civil War letters exhibit many of the symptoms detailed in the modern-day DSM. Correspondence is one of the primary ways historians can gain insight into the psyche of the Civil War solider and those who served in other capacities during the war. From wives to friends and other family members, letters were a critical resource connecting soldiers to something other than the realities and horrors of war. Whether relating a family story or reminiscing about a home-cooked meal, letters were the bridge to life before the war. If a soldier was fortunate, he would receive a package from home that included delicious treats that could be shared with the camp.[125]

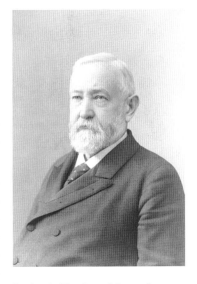

Benjamin Harrison. *Library of Congress, Washington, D.C.*

Another source of entertainment for soldiers was the dime novel. Civil War soldiers read dime novels voraciously, passing them from man to man until the books fell apart. The short books tell stories of adventure and courage through characters such as Frank Reade and Buffalo Bill. Famous abolitionist William Wells Brown entered the dime novel arena with his character Clotel and the series *Books for Camp Fires.*

From a practical standpoint, soldiers purchased paper, ink, pens and envelopes from stationery makers, who engraved the writing materials with various scenes that evoked patriotic feelings in the writer and the reader.[126] Sometimes envelopes were elaborately decorated for a particular regiment.[127]

In the beginning of the war, soldiers paid for stamps and postage to mail letters at post offices near camp. Mail service would track the movements of a regiment. However, as the war progressed, organizations like the U.S. Sanitary Commission gave away paper and envelopes to Union soldiers for free, and in 1864, the U.S. Mail Service permitted soldiers to send letters home for free if they wrote the words "Soldier's Letter" on the outside of the correspondence. You will notice some of the letters published in this book contain misspellings and incorrect word usage. This was due in no small measure to the fact that many soldiers lacked formal education or had attained only a limited level of formal education. Despite the misspellings, soldiers conveyed the trauma and fear they experienced during wartime.[128]

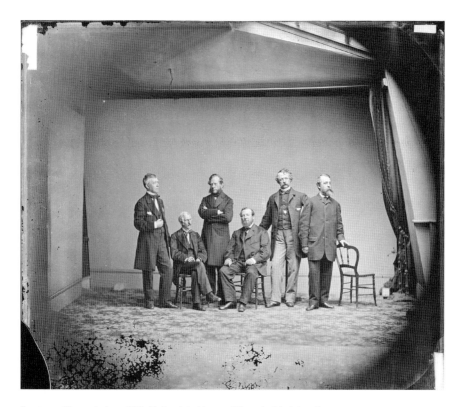

Sanitary Commission. *U.S. National Archives and Records Administration.*

A letter from Thomas Donahue of New York, a Union soldier in the First New York Light Artillery (Pettit's Battery), written from Warrentown, Virginia, to Almira Winchell in Onondaga, New York, on October 29, 1863, reads:[129]

> *Warrenton Va Oct 29th/1863*
> *Friend Almira*
>
> *I will now answer your kind letter which I received the 24 & was very Glad to hear from you and to hear that you was all well I was Sorry to hear that lettie and Gusta had been So Sick but I am Glad to hear that they are better I am well and enjoying myself as well as Can be expected Down here in Dixie I tell you we have had Some very hard marching lately from Culpeper to Centreville is about "60" miles and now we are going Back the Same road we Came on last week we Crossed the old bull run battle Field and we Could See lots of Skeletons of men that were killed there a year ago and were left on top of the if I had been to home and See that I would think it awful but to See a dead man here why it haint nothing I have Seen dead Rebels at the Battle of Antietam lay right in the road and the wheels of the Guns would run over them and the boys would let them lay there you Spoke about John Jones I know that he is not back to his Regiment because I Saw them the other day the boys is all well John Brown is fatter than a hog I Saw bill brown about a week ago he is well he was over to our Camp and I and Ed House had quite a long talk with him you Spoke about the men that was drafted well that is all right enough but I would a little rather they would keep that 900 off and make the men Come and help end this accursed war I See that old abe has Called for three hundred thousand more men I Guess that Some of them will have to Come out here yet and do a little Something for their Country well I Guess I have written enough So I will Close Excuse all mistakes and poor writing my love to all write Soon I remain ever your Friend*
> *Thomas Donahue Almira Pettits Battery*
> *Reserve artillery Army of Potomac*
> *Almira Thomas*

In this letter, Donahue speaks of seeing dead soldiers lying in the road and talks of how common a sight it was for him and others. He then continues the letter in a fairly matter-of-fact manner. Emotional numbness and repression are hallmarks of trauma and PTSD and may be part of how Donahue coped with his nightmarish circumstances.

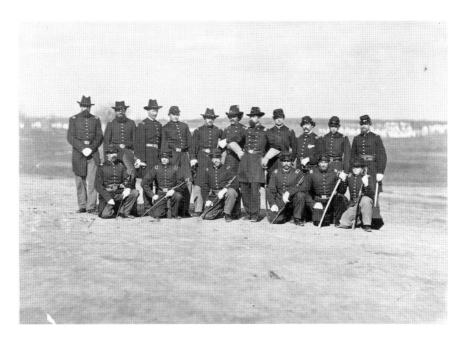

Officers of the Forty-Fourth New York Infantry. *Library of Congress, Washington, D.C.*

Some soldiers took the physical and mental wartime trauma and used their experiences to revolutionize the medical field. J.E. Hanger, credited as the first amputee of the Civil War, is one such example. On June 3, 1861, eighteen-year-old James Edward Hanger was a Confederate private guarding the Baltimore and Ohio Railroad when he was shot in the leg near the knee joint. Union scouts found him, and Dr. James D. Robinson of the Sixteenth Ohio Infantry amputated the young man's leg. Hanger was a prisoner of war until his release in August 1861. He returned home and invented a prosthetic leg, the Hanger Limb. He conceived several designs before receiving his first U.S. Patent on February 14, 1871. His business moved to Washington, D.C., in 1888.[130]

One group's role that often gets overlooked during the Civil War era is the service of Chinese soldiers and sailors. Their stories of trauma, valor and courage are crucial. According to author Stuart Heaver:

> *Prior to the California gold rush, Chinese sailors, cooks and stewards served on ships plying their trade between the Pearl River Estuary and the eastern seaboard of America. Many of these seafarers settled in east coast ports such as New York, a city built largely on the spoils of this lucrative*

China trade. In 1856, a New York Times article headlined "Chinamen in New York" estimated that there were about 150 Chinese men living in lower Manhattan, "mostly employed as sailors." Corporal John Tommy served in Company D, 70th New York Infantry at Gettysburg. Despite the simple Western name foisted on him, he was a native of China. He lost all four limbs on July 2, 1863, and died of his wounds on October 19.

To many, it seemed that slavery had been defeated only to be replaced with denigrating low-cost "coolie labour" that looked remarkably similar. One Chinese veteran who did manage to obtain US citizenship was Hang. Naturalised in New York on October 6, 1892, he voted at every subsequent election until August 17, 1904, when he was arrested while exercising his franchise. Producing his papers, Hang was then subjected to a tirade by an assistant US attorney, who accused the issuing judge of "inexcusable ignorance." On October 21, 1908, New York's Supreme Court set aside his hard-earned citizenship."

Nobody knows the Chinese name of John Tommy or John Tomney as he was also known but he was mentioned in several newspapers in both North and South because he became a Confederate prisoner of war in 1862. He'd enlisted at the age of 18, a new immigrant not knowing much, if any, English at all, in the 70th Regiment New York Infantry on May 15, 1861, one month to the day after the war started. He must have learned the language fast though because he quickly became known as a great wit in camp.

In May 1862 he was captured by the Confederates in Virginia. The capture of a "Chinaman" was mentioned in both Fredericksburg and Richmond newspapers although they didn't name him. In an additional detail supplied by the chaplain of the 4th Texas Regiment the captured "Celestial" was an uncooperative prisoner and was beaten. If so, the beating had remarkably little effect on Tommy. As the New York World of July 9, 1863 reported, "He was brought before Gen. Magruder who, surprised at his appearance and color, asked him was he a mulatto, Indian, or what? When Tommy told him he was from China, Magruder was very much amused, and asked him how much he would take to join the Confederate army. 'Not unless you would make me a Brigadier General.' said Tommy, to the great delight of the secesh officers, who treated him very kindly and sent him to Fredericksburg." He was eventually transferred to the notorious Libby Prison in Richmond, Virginia where overcrowding and unsanitary conditions led to high death rates among the prisoners. Tommy was eventually paroled and spent his recovery time in New York City caring for sick and wounded soldiers and keeping their spirits up.

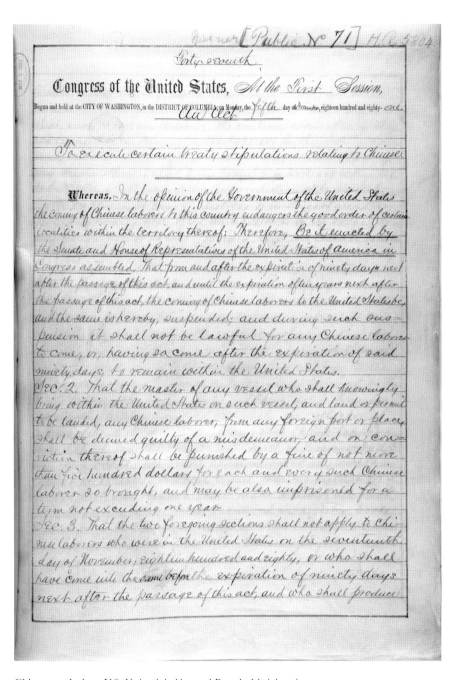

Chinese exclusion. *U.S. National Archives and Records Administration.*

John Tommy later rejoined his regiment and quite remarkably in an otherwise all-white regiment was promoted to corporal; a measure of the respect he must have earned from his fellow soldiers and their officers. He fought in the bloody Battles of Fredericksburg, Chancellorsville, and finally at the most famous battle of the Civil War, Gettysburg. His company, with a normal paper strength of around 80–100 men, went into action already reduced to just 28 men, 20 of whom ended up dead or wounded at Gettysburg. Among the dead was Corporal John Tommy after he'd lost both his legs to cannon fire and bled to death on July 3rd. President Lincoln later dedicated his Gettysburg Address to soldiers such as John Tommy who gave their lives that

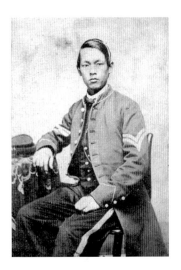

Joseph Pierce. *National Parks Service.*

their nation might live and famously resolved, "...that these dead shall not have died in vain—that this nation, under God, shall have a new birth of freedom—and that government of the people, by the people, for the people, shall not perish from the earth."[131]

SERGEANT CORNELIUS V. MOORE OF COMPANY B, 100TH NEW YORK VOLUNTEERS[132]

Cornelius V. Moore was twenty years old when he enlisted as a Union soldier in the Civil War, joining the 100th New York Infantry alongside his elder brother Edward Moore. An artist by occupation, he kept a record of his and Edward's service during the war through illustrated letters sent home to another brother, Henry, in envelopes with elaborately lettered addresses.[133] "I hope you will find out whether we got to stay 3 years or 9 months," Cornelius writes in a letter dated January 13, 1863, shortly after he enlisted. Cornelius and Edward were stationed at Morris Island, South Carolina, which the former would later describe as having "no trees, nothing but white sand."[134]

Cornelius's letter of March 5, 1863, shows that romantic drama reached the men at war in the Deep South. "Ed got the Valentine but you must

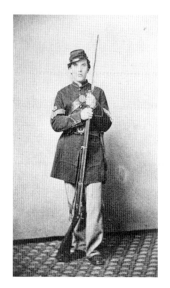

Cornelius Moore. *Library of Congress, Washington, D.C.*

not say anything about it," he writes. "It had Sarah's name on it. I did not read that letter which Sarah sent Ed but Ed read it and said that he would not answer it."

The Moores' company was detached from the regiment, so they could avoid picket duty. "We don't have any thing to do but to paint," reports a grateful Cornelius, who also included a wry sketch of an incoming cannonball threatening to knock over the paint cans. The summer and fall passed with little incident for the Moores. "Every thing is quiet down here," notes Cornelius on December 22. The men were still in the dark about the service they owed. "If you hear anything about it let us know. The talk in camp is that the regiment will be in Buffalo by the 4th of July. We can't tell how true it is." Cornelius had to resort to asking his family for enlistment news. The rumors were false. Cornelius's letter of November 27, 1864, brought news of a sharp change in the men's fates. They were both taken prisoner at Drewry's Bluff, Virginia, on May 16. Cornelius was taken to infamous Andersonville, Georgia. For the first four months, including a twenty-two-day stretch of rain, he and his fellow prisoners were kept in a stockade, with "no shelter but the Heavens above us." Rations consisted of a piece of cornbread, a square inch of pork and occasionally a few spoonfuls of rice. Edward had been sent to the prison at Milan, Georgia. Forced to subsist under equal or worse conditions, he died on October 29, 1864. Disease was the culprit in the official record; exhaustion and starvation were the reason in Cornelius's account.

Cornelius was paroled on November 20. "I thought I would never see you again but there is hope now," he writes joyously to his family.

By March 1865, Cornelius had returned to the 100th New York, now stationed at Richmond, Virginia, in the 24th Corps of the Army of the James. That winter, Cornelius was promoted twice, to corporal and then sergeant, and his corps enjoyed an increase in rations and the respect of officers and soldiers from both armies. A Rebel soldier, noticing that the badge of the 24th Corps was emblazoned with a heart, remarked to Cornelius that "hearts was trumps." Even General Robert E. Lee, according to one of Cornelius's letters home, "said that Grant could be well proud of the 24th corps." After

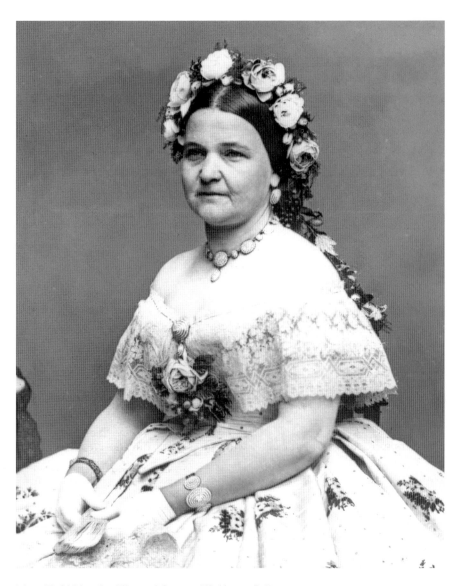

Mary Todd Lincoln. *Library of Congress, Washington, D.C.*

the Confederate surrender, Cornelius Moore and his comrades received heroes' welcomes back into Richmond. He describes the scene in a letter on April 24: "The soldiers that was in Richmond was all formed in line along the gutters of the side walk to receive us. They played the bands of every reg't as we walk by them. It was nice to see the folks in Richmond and the stores all open selling everything."

Letter between Cornelius Moore and Stanton. *Library of Congress, Washington, D.C.*

The corps dutifully waited for the repair of the railroad that would take them to Washington and eventually home. But nothing happened quickly. Three months after the surrender and the fanfare in Richmond, Cornelius was still in Virginia with his regiment—though with another promotion, to first sergeant. Still seeking an answer to the question he had been asking for two years, Moore wrote to Secretary of War Edwin Stanton, requesting an honorable discharge.[135]

"I entered the service when the government needed the services of its loyal citizens, to maintain its integrity, suppress secession and ensure its permanency," he asserts. But the war's end had made fighting for these ideals no longer necessary, and Cornelius felt he had fulfilled his duty in his months of suffering "all the horrors of Andersonville," his brother's death and his dedication to his regiment in its subsequent occupation of Richmond. "The service…owing to its inactivity has become onerous to me," he admits.

Perhaps Stanton intervened. Either way, Cornelius Moore, "Occupation: Artist" written in intricate lettering, was finally discharged from the U.S. Army on August 28, 1865.[136]

The Andersonville Prison diary of Alfred H. Voorhees, Company H, First New York Cavalry gives a painful yet unique window into the traumatic life

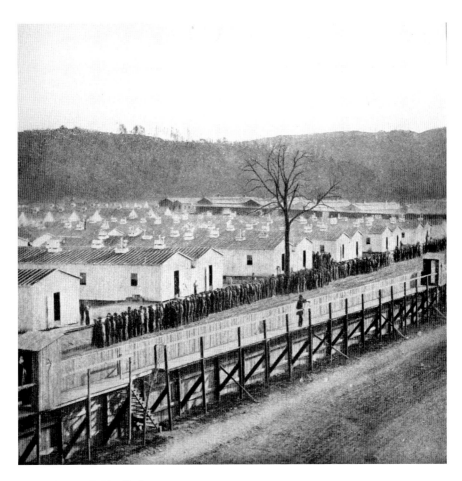

Elmira Prison. *Wikimedia Commons.*

of prisoners. On May 25, 1864, Voorhees writes, "Arrived at Andersonville today, the place of our destination. See quite a number of my [regiment] here a hard place it is too, the boys ruff, all kinds of huts and shanties. Some have been here 8 months. Feel a good deal better a day, a close, 18,000. Men on 10 acres."[137]

On May 29, 1864, according to Voorhees, "More prisoners arrived today, the Prison is crowded full. Don't know what they will do with any more. How different from home and sabbath [comforts], all we can see is filth and dirt. All combined makes it a hard, lingering place. Some die, poor fellows from 30 to 40 per day. Hope I will live through this and see home once more."[138]

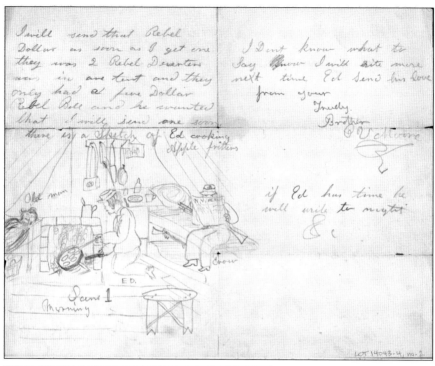

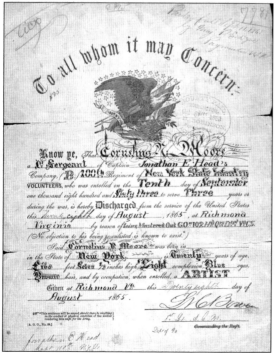

Above: Cornelius Moore letter. *Library of Congress, Washington, D.C.*

Left: Cornelius Moore letter. *Library of Congress, Washington, D.C.*

Opposite: Letter between Cornelius Moore and Stanton. *Library of Congress, Washington, D.C.*

C. Moore, was also taken prisoner at the same time and died from exhaustion and Starvation at Millen, Ga, prison in October, 1864,

Returning to duty in February, I was with my regiment up to the occupation of Richmond, and have won promotion for soldierly behavior in discharge of duty,

Having faithfully discharged my duty I my health being impaired by suffering and fatigues incident to my imprisonment, and the treatment I received, I most respectfully request the honorable Secretary to grant me an honorable discharge from the service, which, owing to its inactivity has become onerous to me, Your favorable consideration and reply will be gratefully received, and remembered by Your

Obedient Servt.
C. N. Moore -
orderly Sergt. Co B. 100th N.Y. Vols,
24th Army Corks. Brig Gen Dandy Brig

On May 30, 1864, Voorhees's situation is made very clear in his diary entry:

> *This is hell on earth today and yesterday. More Yanks came today so thick one can scarcely walk. A number of the boys go out to work on the stockade to enlarge the Prison. Don't feel well today. Some talk of a parole soon. Can't feed us with proper food. Oh that we may soon be relieved but we must wait hoping we will not get sick.* [139]

Voorhees died on August 13, 1864.

Made famous by Ken Burns during the PBS series *The Civil War*, this letter from Sullivan Ballou to his wife is a good manifestation of the pain and loss that so many soldiers experienced:

> *July the 14th, 1861*
> *Washington DC*
>
> *My very dear Sarah:*
>
> *The indications are very strong that we shall move in a few days—perhaps tomorrow. Lest I should not be able to write you again, I feel impelled to write lines that may fall under your eye when I shall be no more.*
>
> *Our movement may be one of a few days duration and full of pleasure—and it may be one of severe conflict and death to me. Not my will, but thine O God, be done. If it is necessary that I should fall on the battlefield for my country, I am ready. I have no misgivings about, or lack of confidence in, the cause in which I am engaged, and my courage does not halt or falter. I know how strongly American Civilization now leans upon the triumph of the Government, and how great a debt we owe to those who went before us through the blood and suffering of the Revolution. And I am willing—perfectly willing—to lay down all my joys in this life, to help maintain this Government, and to pay that debt.*
>
> *But, my dear wife, when I know that with my own joys I lay down nearly all of yours, and replace them in this life with cares and sorrows—when, after having eaten for long years the bitter fruit of orphanage myself, I must offer it as their only sustenance to my dear little children—is it weak or dishonorable, while the banner of my purpose floats calmly and proudly in the breeze, that my unbounded love for you, my darling wife and children, should struggle in fierce, though useless, contest with my love of country?*

I cannot describe to you my feelings on this calm summer night, when two thousand men are sleeping around me, many of them enjoying the last, perhaps, before that of death—and I, suspicious that Death is creeping behind me with his fatal dart, am communing with God, my country, and thee.

I have sought most closely and diligently, and often in my breast, for a wrong motive in thus hazarding the happiness of those I loved and I could not find one. A pure love of my country and of the principles have often advocated before the people and "the name of honor that I love more than I fear death" have called upon me, and I have obeyed.

Sarah, my love for you is deathless, it seems to bind me to you with mighty cables that nothing but Omnipotence could break; and yet my love of Country comes over me like a strong wind and bears me irresistibly on with all these chains to the battlefield.

The memories of the blissful moments I have spent with you come creeping over me, and I feel most gratified to God and to you that I have enjoyed them so long. And hard it is for me to give them up and burn to ashes the hopes of future years, when God willing, we might still have lived and loved together and seen our sons grow up to honorable manhood around us. I have, I know, but few and small claims upon Divine Providence, but something whispers to me—perhaps it is the wafted prayer of my little Edgar—that I shall return to my loved ones unharmed. If I do not, my dear Sarah, never forget how much I love you, and when my last breath escapes me on the battlefield, it will whisper your name.

Forgive my many faults, and the many pains I have caused you. How thoughtless and foolish I have oftentimes been! How gladly would I wash out with my tears every little spot upon your happiness, and struggle with all the misfortune of this world, to shield you and my children from harm. But I cannot. I must watch you from the spirit land and hover near you, while you buffet the storms with your precious little freight, and wait with sad patience till we meet to part no more.

But, O Sarah! If the dead can come back to this earth and flit unseen around those they loved, I shall always be near you; in the garish day and in the darkest night—amidst your happiest scenes and gloomiest hours—always, always; and if there be a soft breeze upon your cheek, it shall be my breath; or the cool air fans your throbbing temple, it shall be my spirit passing by.

Sarah, do not mourn me dead; think I am gone and wait for thee, for we shall meet again.

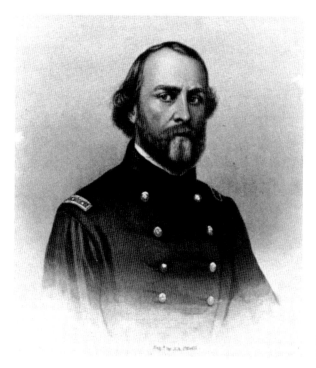

Sullivan Ballou.
Wikimedia Commons.

As for my little boys, they will grow as I have done, and never know a father's love and care. Little Willie is too young to remember me long, and my blue eyed Edgar will keep my frolics with him among the dimmest memories of his childhood. Sarah, I have unlimited confidence in your maternal care and your development of their characters. Tell my two mothers his and hers I call God's blessing upon them. O Sarah, I wait for you there! Come to me, and lead thither my children.[140]

What makes this letter so impactful from a trauma standpoint? First, the letter is infused with the uncertainty that soldiers inevitably experience during war. From when he and his comrades will leave camp to what his future will look like, Ballou's uncertainty is palpable. This is a key ingredient for trauma.

Next, loneliness and Ballou speaking poignantly about how much he misses his "Dear Sarah" and how difficult the wartime is without her.

Third, longing for home and what has been left behind. Ballou reminisces about cherished "memories" and how they wash over him. This level of disconnectedness from home can be excruciatingly stressful at any time, but with the added horror of war, it can be almost unbearable.

Some letters soldiers wrote are illustrative mainly because of how they show the homesickness many felt. This, as the book discusses, is an important factor in an overall trauma picture. This letter from Francis M. Russell is one such example:

Washington City, D.C. Sunday, Dec. 14th 1862

Dear Mother and family,

I will take the pensil to let you know we are all well. At present hoping this will find you in the same. we let White Hall Station on Thursday about 4 Clock in the afternoon and got into Washington about 4 oclock in the morning on Friday whitch maid about 12 hours on the way, we then stay ther untill yesterday when we had orders to march about 6.5 miles and when I heard this I went to the head doctor ast him what I would do for I know that I could not carry my knapsack, so he told me that I would have to stay hear and so all them that could not stand the march was sent to the hospitle. Ther was 10 out of our Company and that was myself and a nother young man, we did not hear the name of the place that they wer going to, but both James and Bob said that they would wright as soon as they wer sitteled that is they would wright home to you, ther is abut 50 sick and wounded in the department that I am in, I think that I will not be in hear very long, for I will try and get eather home or get to my Regiment for I don't like this very well, it is not because I am not treated well for it is six times better than I expected but I canot be contented a way from my companny, my arm is about the same, I wright this mearley to let you know something about myselve for I canot say anything about the others now but I will have to stope so no more at present but reman your son and Brother.
Francis M. Russell
Address your letter to Stanton Hosepittle, Washington City. C.C.
I wish you would send me some postige stamps as we have not got paid yet, my money has run ashore and I want to wright some and so on.
Yours, F.M.R.

The interesting aspects of Russell's letter are that, besides the loneliness he described, the content notes the importance of payday and how this could impact the mental health of a soldier. As he had not yet been paid, Russell needed money in order to write more letters to his family. As stated elsewhere in the book, writing and reading letters were crucial activities for

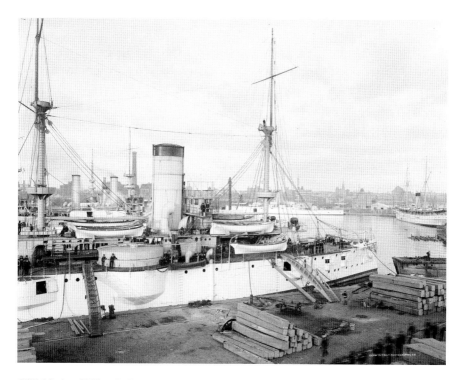

CSS *Monitor. Wikimedia Commons.*

many soldiers. Russell's letter also speaks to the intersection of physical and psychological symptoms, which seems to be in part why he found himself hospitalized. "Payday was wonderful for soldiers. In addition to having funds to send to loved ones, soldiers were able to indulge in treats for themselves that made the work go somewhat faster. From fresh fruits and foods to getting additional provisions and simply being able to spend time with comrades in a relaxed fashion, leisure time for the soldiers was welcome indeed."[141]

Lewis Brave Jr., born on December 20, 1840, enlisted in the army on December 1, 1861, in the Regimental Band of the Twelfth New York Volunteer Infantry Regiment. He was mustered out on July 19, 1862. In a passage from his diary, he listed some provisions he and his companions received: "This morning we got our stoves, tin plates, spoons, knives and forks, coffee pot, wash dish, camp kettle, dish pan, tin pail and pork, rice, beans, sugar, coffee, bread and salt."[142] These were important items to soldiers, a fact not lost to healthcare workers such as Clara Barton.

Senator Henry Wilson of Massachusetts and Clara Barton were friends. Both were from Massachusetts and Wilson served as something of a champion for Barton and her efforts, so a letter like the one that follows would not have been unusual for her to write. In it, she desperately requested necessary supplies for the soldiers in her care. Barton was sensitive to the psychological impact lack of supplies had on the soldiers and how it added to the suffering of those soldiers

Washington, D.C. January 18, 1863
Hon. H. Wilson
U.S. Senator

Sir: I take the liberty to request that you would assist me to procure through the Surgeon General such a supply of medical store as I can use successfully on the battle field or in the hospital. Any transportation or commissary stores are kindly and readily supplied me by Col. Rucker. Dr. Hammond also furnished me some months ago a fine lot of liquors which were mainly at Fredericksburg. The last cup I remember to have distributed among the poor sufferers who were shot in Saturday's fight and left dying upon the field, until brought across the river under flag of truce on Tuesday night (the little clothing left on them saturated in blood and frozen firmly to them) most of them in chills and cramps to be lain upon the ground (in tents) with light covering and no fires. I shall never forget my own gratitude to say nothing of theirs for the possession of the little comforts I held in store for them.

The articles I most need at present are whiskey, brandy, wine, condensed milk, prepared meats, cups, plates, a few dishes and kettles necessary for the preparation of suitable food for sick men, some flannel underclothing and a few blankets.

Feeling assured from the deep and abiding interest I know you to cherish on behalf of our wounded and suffering heroes, I respectfully ask that you would if possible so arrange the matter that I could have permission or an order to draw articles desired from the medical purveyor from time to time as I may need them. You have, I hope, a sufficient assurance of their being prudently and properly applied. If I were able to purchase these things at my own cost I would not ask them of the government. This my circumstances forbid, or if I were able to sit quietly down in the midst of all the suffering and desolation around me without even attempting to relieve any portion of it, then I would not ask. This my attire forbids and hence I just trouble others with my requests.[143]

Disease was the true equalizer during the Civil War. Because of the lack of understanding about why soldiers died in such environments, infections killed many soldiers, as did horrible wounds caused by the Minié ball and other weapons, amputations, disease and lack of medical supplies. This all served to instill in many soldiers both fear of surgery itself as well as life after procedures.[144]

One of the complications for soldiers living without limbs involved their employability after the war. Many soldiers who entered the war had come from lives where their work involved physical labor. Dock work, farming and railroad work were all physically arduous and taxing on the body. Postwar employment for soldiers in certain socioeconomic sets without limbs was scarce, and this was not an era prone to making accommodations for the unique needs of such soldiers. In addition to the physical impact that this disability had both on the soldiers and their families, the psychological stress is undeniable.[145] Comfort is an important aspect of psychological well-being. The ability to be physically close to loved ones as well as comforts such as food, warmth, housing and water all played an important role in the psychological well-being of soldiers and others during the war. Removal of these important items made a difficult situation nearly unbearable for some.[146] "Food supplies were frequently limited and insufficient for the amount of calories a soldier would expel. The water was often contaminated with germs making soldiers sick. Septic water is especially dangerous because it carries many diseases like cholera and dysentery."[147]

Author Sarah Ford notes another interesting factor that led to psychological issues. Soldiers sometimes came from small towns where they knew everyone, including others who were fighting. An entire family might be part of the wartime effort, either fighting on the same side or, more psychologically difficult, on the opposite side.

Active psychological tactics were not uncommon in the Civil War. The Rebel Yell was a weapon used to instill fear in the Union soldiers. Confederate soldiers would yell, shout or chant certain phrases or noises to frighten their enemies, and many times it did its job. The sounds were described variously as whooping noises and the shrieks of a wild animal, terrifying the soldiers: "[T]he Union troops were startled by the most hideous of modern war cries, known as the 'rebel yell.'…This was the first time the Vermont boys had heard that fiendish sound, and it is not too much to say that they were appalled by it for a moment, and thought their time had come to be 'wiped out.'"[148]

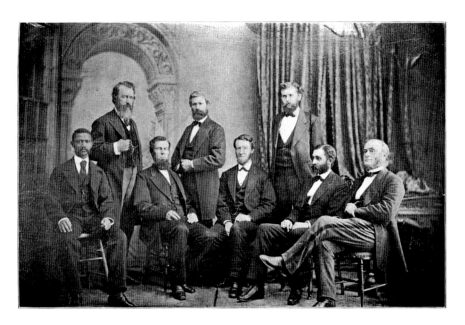

Howard University faculty, 1860s. *National Library of Medicine.*

Hand-to-hand combat has been identified as a leading cause of trauma experienced by soldiers during war. From utilizing bayonets at close range to actually being in sustained physical contact with another enemy soldier, hand-to-hand combat seems to have played an extraordinarily detrimental role in the psyche of soldiers from this period.[149] Adding to the trauma experienced by soldiers during the war were the conditions. According to Julia Wheelock, who worked in Washington, D.C.–area hospitals in the 1860s, there were ten thousand wounded in Fredericksburg, Virginia.[150] "All the public buildings, including the courthouse, churches, hotels, warehouses, factories, paper mill, theater, school buildings, stores, stables, and private residences were converted into shelters for the wounded, until Fredericksburg was one vast hospital."[151]

Wheelock recalled soldiers desperately requesting pillows: "I'm wounded in the head, and my knapsack is so hard," said one. Another wanted one for his stump. "I don't think it would be so painful if I only had a pillow, or cushion, or something to keep it from the hard floor," the soldier bemoaned.[152] Additionally,

> One "wretched hospital," a former grocery store, had only a single small candle for light. When someone moved the candle to another part of the

crowded room, Wheelock, afraid she would stumble over the injured, crept on her hands and knees to deliver cups of broth to the wounded, starving soldiers. Many were so fresh from the battlefield that their wounds were still undressed. Given such conditions, it was small wonder that the often overwhelmed military medical establishment could not care adequately for victims with poorly understood psychological needs.[153]

Suicide was another tragic consequence both during the war and once soldiers and others involved in the war returned home. Soldiers wrote to family and friends about others who had taken their lives and the level of despondency experienced by their comrades. Despite not having the medical training to diagnose a fellow soldier, many could easily see the psychological pain their friends were experiencing because they were experiencing it themselves.[154]

Solutions for widows were important as well. In an unprecedented move, Lincoln allowed a black woman, the widow of Civil War soldier Major Lionel F. Booth, to meet with him at the White House. Mary Booth's husband had been killed at Fort Pillow, Tennessee, in April 1864 by a Confederate sniper. The massacre of African American Union forces that followed the subsequent fall of the fort was considered one of the most brutal of the Civil War. After speaking with Mrs. Booth privately, Lincoln sat down and wrote a letter of introduction for her to carry to Sumner asking him to hear what she had to say about the hardships imposed on families of black soldiers killed or maimed in battle. The letter introduced Booth's widow, stating that her important focus on widows and children of African American soldiers should receive the same benefits as other soldiers.

As a result of his meeting with Mrs. Booth, in 1866, Senator Sumner influenced congressional members to introduce a resolution (H.R. 406, Section 13) to provide for the equal treatment of the dependents of African American soldiers.

A 2006 study of military and Pension Board medical records of 17,700 Civil War

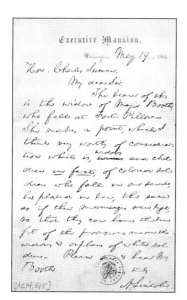

Letter between Lincoln and Sumner. *Library of Congress, Washington, D.C.*

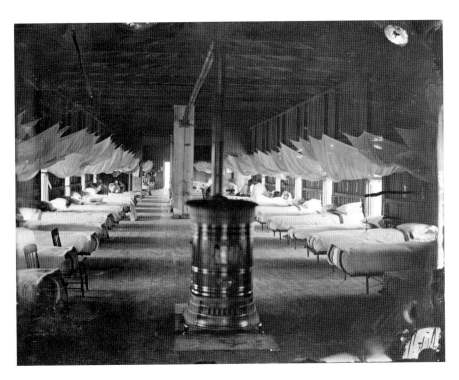

Harewood General Hospital. *Wikimedia Commons.*

veterans found an association between the men's wartime experiences and the occurrence of cardiac, gastrointestinal and nervous diseases throughout the remainder of their lives. One measure found a 51 percent increase in those three disease categories. Those removed from the battlefield were marked by their experiences as well. A civilian relief worker wrote that after the Battles of the Wilderness and Spotsylvania, "The surgeons were at work, probing, extracting balls, amputating in the open air, while upon every hand were cries of agony from the poor fellows, which would have melted any but a heart of stone." Years later, Nurse Lois Dunbar recalled, "I have had men die clutching my dress till it was almost impossible to lose their hold." Even experienced doctors and nurses could not easily forget such sights and sounds.[155] Another hallmark of those suffering from trauma is shame. Civil War veterans deliberately hid their trauma affliction for fear of losing pensions. Second to that was secondary trauma and pain that families experienced during the war. This letter from Captain Squire speaks eloquently of secondary trauma and pain that families experienced during the war, with Squire spending a fair amount of time comforting his parents and the pain they expressed in separate letters to him. Squire speaks about the war effort generally in his letter below and then spends a fair amount of time lamenting over the pain the war caused his family.

Captain Watson Squire letter to his parents May 21, 1861

Elmira NY May 21, 1861 Dear father and mother, Your letters have both been received. I was much grieved at the sad tone of both. Of course we all deprecate war. But since the question of our existence as a nation seems to hang upon a thread, and in case a dissolution takes place war is inevitable. I say let us come when we are best prepared and when we have the national prestige and resources to back US. Who wishes to see a reenaction of the Mexican feuds. There if a party fails in a presidential election it immediately sets up in opposition and usually so with success. What is our government good for if it cannot maintain itself. If the people are to rule in any locality they must do it by majorities. And if it those majorities are to be successfully set a defiance by then the experiment of self-government is at an end. I say we have a greater cause for which to battle, now than did our revolutionary sites. They fought against taxation without representation we fight for the doctrine of self-government. Acquiescence in the demands of the South would be next to disintegration of the whole nation. The irremediable disgrace for us all and feeling of despair in the breasts of freeman all over the globe. There is no knowing where the consequences of such a step would end. We should see European tragedies of state aced over on the American soil. What can be done to arrest this lava tide of woe? Nothing but a firm resistance to rebellion can save us. Instead of creating wars we shall diminish and mitigate them by a united overpowering effort to maintain the government. It is successful then indeed will the world with shouts of delight, and it not so, we at least save and bind together with everlasting bonds that band of states, which adhere to the general government.

But I will not dwell longer upon a discussion of these wars. I have not much time to write now but the tone of your letters grieved me so much that I felt I must write something immediately. I think you are too much concerned about me. I am very glad to have those who care for me, but I can not bear to have their bosoms rent with anguish. If there could have been anything that would have deterred me from the course I have chosen it would be the thought of plunging my parents into affliction. I appreciate all you have done for me. I shall try to be a faithful steward of what you have

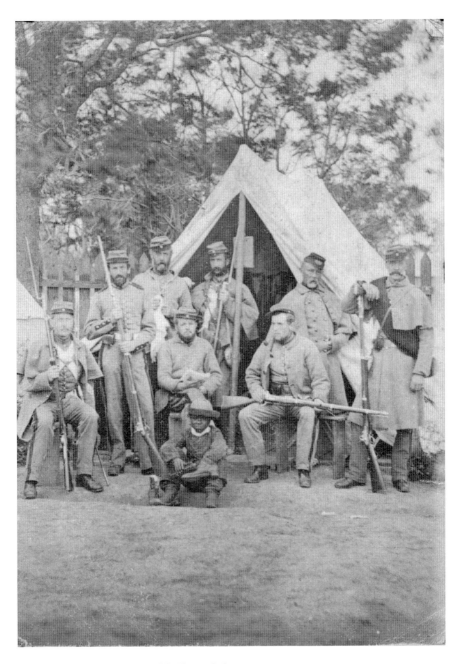

Camp life. *Library of Congress, Washington, D.C.*

bestowed upon me. Of course we none of us know that chances of war. I may return with honor and invigorated constitution. I hope by a prudent course so to do. Camp life thus far has been as easy for me as for any that are with me. We have had no camp, but rather a life in the barracks.

The stories of veterans after the war are compelling in nature and scope. There's the story of Emerson Clark, who died at the age of ninety-two and was the last G.A.R. veteran in Putnam County, New York. According to the *Putnam County Courier* of Carmel, New York, Clark enlisted in the war on January 13, 1864, as a private of Company B, Sixteenth New York Heavy Artillery. He mustered out on August 21, 1865, in Washington, D.C. Clark was born in Chatham, New York, on August 10, 1848, and recalled that he was anxious to enlist in the war but did in fact enlist as a drummer boy and stated that in his opinion, the rifle was the most dangerous weapon during the war because of the formation of the soldiers. He also spoke about army life and opined that battles were much easier than living in camps. "We ate meat. This 'junk' was boiled up in a large kettle which was caked with salt. It was chopped off in chunks. It tasted like meat but so salted you couldn't tell what it was....Beans were also my favorite. Sleeping, too, had its difficulties."[156] Clark spent many nights in his tent gazing up at the stars. He served for eighteen months and was honorably discharged.[157]

The ability of hospitals to care for veterans with chronic need postwar was spotty. In the summer of 1862, John Hildt lost one of his limbs. The twenty-five-year-old corporal from Michigan saw combat for the first time at the Seven Days Battle in Virginia, where he was shot in the right arm. Doctors amputated his shattered limb close to the shoulder, causing a severe hemorrhage. Hildt survived his physical wounds but was transferred to the government hospital for the insane in Washington, D.C., suffering from acute mania. Hildt, a laborer who'd risen quickly in the ranks, had no prior history of mental illness, and his siblings wrote to the asylum expressing surprise that his mind could not be restored to "its original state."[158] But months and then years passed, without improvement. Hildt remained

Oliver Otis Howard. *U.S. National Archives and Records Administration.*

withdrawn, apathetic and at times so excited and disturbed that he hit other patients at the asylum. He finally died there in 1911.[159]

Jacob Lester was born on June 24, 1847, and died on June 28, 1947. He enlisted in the army on September 17, 1863. On October 10, 1863, he was assigned to Company F, First New York Veteran Calvary. He was promoted to corporal on June 1, 1865. According to the *Binghamton Press*, in an interview with Lester on May 29, 1945, "[He] doesn't need steel in his hand to recall Newmarket or Kernstown or the wild ride up the Shenandoah Valley with the enemy at his heels. Nor has he forgotten the sounds and smells at the hospital in Martinsburg and the sight of a buddy with a bullet hole in his chest."[160]

Lewis Henry Douglass was the oldest son of Frederick Douglass and Anna Murray Douglass. Lewis Henry was born in New Bedford, Massachusetts, and apprenticed as a typesetter at his father's newspaper, *North Star*, and Douglass's weekly. On March 25, 1863, he joined the Union army as a member of the Fifty-Fourth Massachusetts. He was a sergeant major and participated in the famed Battle of Fort Wagner. In a letter to his future wife, Douglass speaks of the horrors and traumas of war:

> *My dear Amelia. This regiment has established its reputation as a fighting regiment not a man flinched, though it was a trying time. Men fell all around me. A shell would explode and clear a space of twenty feet, or men would close up again, but it was no use we had to retreat, which was a very hazardous undertaking.*

Douglas ends his letter to his future wife with hope:

> *How I got out of that fight alive I cannot tell, but I am here. My Dear girl, I hope again to see you. I must bid you farewell should I be killed. Remember if I should die I die in a good cause. I wish we had a hundred thousand colored troops. We would put an end to this war. Good Bye to all. Write soon. Your own loving Lewis.*[161]

Lewis was wounded at Wagner and was discharged from the army in 1864. He eventually settled in Washington, D.C., in 1869 with his wife, Helen Amelia Loguen. Loguen was a Syracuse, New York native, and they married there on October 7, 1869. Lewis Henry Douglass and his father established the *New National Era* paper in 1870. The focus was issues in the D.C. black community. He was appointed to the D.C. legislative council by Ulysses S. Grant.[162]

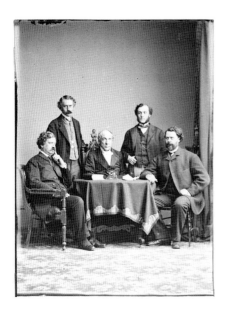

Sanitary Commission. *U.S. National Archives and Records Administration.*

Author and television anchor Cheryl Wills gives an impactful account of Frederick Douglass's imprint on the Civil War, the African American troops who served and the country as a whole:

> *Frederick Douglass, who was born in Talbot County, Maryland, around 1818, was a runaway slave himself. In thunderous speeches, he passionately condemned the institution that he had first-hand knowledge about. When Douglass was about 12 years old, his master's wife broke the law by teaching him the letters of the alphabet. His literacy was the beginning of his liberty. Soon he was able to read newspapers and his eyes confirmed what his heart had always known: slavery was immoral and on its deathbed. After several failed attempts, Douglass successfully ran away from his plantation in September of 1838. After stops throughout the Northeast, he settled in Massachusetts, where he became a prominent abolitionist, agitator, author, and ultimately the most famous black man in America, perhaps in the world. With prominent facial features and a dignified statuesque build, Douglass finally got the ear of President Lincoln.*[163]

Families, Friends and Advocates
in New York and D.C.
during and after the War

The trauma of war extended to family members seeking to locate missing soldiers after the war. Clara Barton was an advocate for many whose loved ones were missing at the end of the hostilities. Countless family members wrote to Barton with tragic tales of not being able to find missing soldiers. In reaction to the outpouring of requests for information, in 1865, Barton founded the Office of Correspondence with Friends of the Missing Men of the United States Army, located in Washington, D.C. She contacted hospitals, newspapers and other localities that might know the whereabouts of soldiers. Congress appropriated $15,000 for the project. Barton and her team responded to over sixty-three thousand letters, locating more than twenty-two thousand soldiers.[164]

Some of these letters are reproduced here.

December 29th 1865

Dear friends

A letter of December 4 asking information of your "son" DH Windham, last heard of at Fort Wagner is before me. Ordinarily, I should reply to your inquiry by saying that I would place the name upon my rolls of missing men, and search as best I could. I will do so—But your letter draws upon my recollections of a few words more. Not that I remember your son, I wish I did, but I remember the charge on Wagner that terrible night at the 18th of July 1863—Only those whose eyes took in that scene will ever realize it. During four long hours preceding that charge, I watched those doomed men marching and counter marching, or fixed in a solid phalanx waiting that charge of death. Then four other hours of carnage such as God grant you may never realize, where the rolling valleys of destruction alone lit up the misty blackness of the night, then they bore the wounded back along the wave washed beach, and the surging ocean sang its solemn requiem for the dead.

There lay by hundreds, wounded and bleeding, in the wet salt sands about my little tent, and God in his goodness gave me speed to my feet and strength to my arms through the hours of that fearful night that I might nourish the fainting slake to staunch the life stream as it ebbed away. It seemed as if daylight would never come, but when at length it's welcome beams broke over us, we were no longer swept by shot, but the field of plaid [upturned] faces and eyes forever still, showed only too plainly how broad a wing the Death Angel had flapped above is, and they told us of a six hundred that lay dead in the Fort, where on no comrade ere might look where of no mother know.

I will not ask your pardon my dear friends for having recalled here events to you—they will neither appease nor distress you, your son was a soldier, his regiment well known to me and you who have suffered so much will be still strong enough to listen while I who stood among, and saw and knew them all, relate the scene which to him I fear were the last of earth—true he may have been captured and a prisoner after this, this I will endeavor by all means in my power to ascertain for you. And I will write to his surgeon, who is my friend, and one of the noblest men in the world, for any clue, which he may give me, and if I can get a trace however I will send it at once to you. Pardon my long letter…truly your friend. Clara Barton.[165]

***

In a poignant letter dated September 26, 1865, Mrs. T.B. Hurlburt of Ripper Alton, Illinois, wrote Barton about her son, Captain Wilbur Hurlburt. He was captain of Company D, Fifth Michigan Infantry. This letter is indicative of many letters written to Barton postwar.

Ripper Alton, Illinois
September 26, 1865
Miss Barton

Dear Madam,

I approach you with my great sorrow, but hardly indulge the hope that you can do anything for me. My darling boy, my only son, was reported killed in the battle of the Wilderness, May 6th 1864. His body was not found and the hope was entertained by his regiment and clutched at by myself, that wounded he had fallen into the hands of, the enemy, a prisoner and not dead. After various fruitless efforts to obtain information, General Longstreet courteously ordered an examination in the southern prisons, and we obtained a certificate from each that no such name had ever been received. After all our investigations we are led to the conclusion that he died on the battlefield, or mortally wounded, was conveyed to some farm house and may have been there been buried....My son was twenty-two years old. Wore no moustache or beard. Was about six feet in height. When in college he was rather spare, but the outdoor life of the army had given him a robust appearance. He entered the army as Aid to General Richardson. After the officer's lamented death, he served in the Michigan Fifth. He had participated in more than twenty battles. Was severely wounded at Gettysburg, but from which he wholly recovered....It may be well to add my son's name to the many missing ones, and could you by any means give to me any knowledge of, the last resting place of my darling one you would confer such a favor as none less desolate than myself can appreciate. May God bless you in your humane efforts and abundantly reward you, Mrs. T.B. Hurlbut, Ripper Alton, Illinois.

P.S. I neglected to mention that my son had dark hazel eyes. Hair almost black.[166]

***

Clara Barton and her good friend Frederick Douglass often shared correspondence regarding postwar assistance for soldiers and their families. One such correspondence involved starting an organization to assist African American women in securing employment postwar. A protracted issue for families and veterans postwar was overall resources. This included a steady income. Many soldiers had physical or mental health issues that precluded them from working in the same manner as they had before the war. It was often left to family members to provide for and ensure the household was managed properly.

My dear Miss Barton:

I am just home from one of those wearing western towns, which I need not describe to you; and find your letter written with a tired hand and at a late hour. Jan: 26. In fulfillment of your promise to write me the result of your interview with General Butler: I sincerely thank you for this letter. It tells me anew, of your devotion to suffering humanity in every form and of every Colour. While in the west, I saw a paper in which it was stated that you have already opened an establishment in Washington to gain employment to destitute colored women willing and able to work. I have seen nothing on the subject since. Your energy, zeal and influence lead me to believe that you are successfully at work. Have you really opened an establishment of any considerable dimensions? Do you find that the result justifies the undertaking? What can I do to help forward the Effort? I hope to be in Washington soon and will there be very glad to see you and learn all about the good work in which you are engaged.

I have come home half sick. My system is much out of joint, but I hope that a few days of the quiet of house will set me all right again.

Believe you how Gen'l Butler as powerful in action as in word. It was a huge undertaking for you to encounter this General and seek to his judgement on the side of your wisely benevolent enterprise and much have been exceedingly gratifying to you, as it certainly is to me, to know.[167]

While this letter focuses on work for African American women, Douglas and Barton often collaborated on issues surrounding civil and women's rights and, in the early 1889s, healthcare, via the creation of the American Branch of the Red Cross. In 1878, Barton published a pamphlet titled "The Red Cross of the Geneva Convention: What It Is" in which she described the Red Cross and the Treaty of Geneva Conference, which "provides for the neutrality of all Sanitary supplies, ambulances, surgeons, nurses, attendants, and the sick or wounded men, and their safe conduct, when they bear this sign of the organization...the Red Cross."[168] One of the benefits of women taking on larger responsibility both in and out of the home were the legal rights they began to accrue. This progress also had residual benefits for overall human rights.

Appeal to the American People

The President having signed the Treaty of the Geneva Conference, and the Senate having, on the 16th instant, ratified President's Action, the American Association of the Red Cross, organized under provisions of said treaty, purposes to send its agents at once among the sufferers by the recent floods, with a view to the ameliorating of their condition so far as can be done by human aid and the means at hand will permit. Contributions are urgently solicited. Remittances in money may be made to Hon. Charles J. Folger, Secretary of the Treasury, Chairman of the Board of Trustees, or to his associates, Hon. Robert T. Lincoln, Secretary of War, and Hon. George B. Loring, Commissioner of Agriculture. Contributions of wearing apparel, bedding and provisions, should be addressed to the Red Cross Agent at Memphis, Tenn., Vicksburg, Miss., and Helena, Ark. Clara Barton, JC Bancroft Davis, Frederick Douglass, Alex Y.P. Garnett, Mrs. Omar D. Conger, A.S. Salomons, Mrs. S.A. Martha Canfield, RD Mussey, Committ and, Washington, D.C. March 23, 1882.

Robert Gould Shaw and the Seventh New York Regiment

Robert Gould Shaw was born in Boston on October 10, 1837. His parents were Francis George Shaw and Sarah Blake Shaw. They were abolitionists, and Unitarians and a fairly wealthy family. In 1847, the family moved to Staten Island, New York. Shaw attended boarding school in the 1850s and then in 1856 enrolled at Harvard. He was a member of the Porcellian Club and the Hasty Pudding Club but left the school in 1859 before graduating. He returned to Staten Island in 1859 and worked at Henry P. Sturgis and Company Mercantile Firm. On April 19, 1861, Shaw joined the Seventh New York Militia. These early letters show the pain, heartache and loneliness that Shaw experienced. They also show the transformation of a young soldier into an iconic hero. Shaw would later go on to fame as the colonel of the Fifty-Fourth Massachusetts Infantry, an all–African American regiment whose bravery is chronicled in the 1989 film *Glory*, starring Matthew

HEALING CIVIL WAR VETERANS IN NEW YORK AND WASHINGTON, D.C.

Broderick, Denzel Washington, Morgan Freeman and Cary Elwes. These early letters portray a somewhat different, but important, Shaw.

On April 18, 1861, Robert Gould Shaw composed letters from his family's Staten Island farm. The Seventh New York had been ordered to Washington on short notice, and Shaw could not properly say goodbye to his family. As it was the beginning of the war, Shaw's letters are filled with the hope of a speedy end to the conflict. It is also interesting to note the different tone with which Shaw writes to his various family members.

North Shore S.I.
Thursday, April 18, 1861

Dearest Mother,

You will probably know when you get this, that the only piece of bad news to greet you when you arrive is that of my departure with the 7th Regt. for Washington. It is very hard to go off without bidding you goodbye, and the only thing that upsets me, in the least, is the thought of how you will feel when you find me so unexpectedly gone.

We all feel that if we can get into Washington, before Virginia begins to make trouble, we shall not have much fighting. We expect to get there on Saturday [April 20].... Won't it be grand to meet the men from all the States, East and West, down there, ready to fight for the country, as the old fellows did in the Revolution?

Our Col. [Marshall Lefferts] tells us we are only going to Washington for the present and shall be sent back to New York as soon as troops from the more distant States can arrive. I feel as if I were not going on anything but an ordinary journey. I can't help crying a little through when I think of Father & you & the girls. Don't be too anxious. Please be careful of your health. May God bless you all. When we are all at home together again, may peace & happiness be restored to the Country. The war has already done us good, in making the North so united.

Shaw's letter to his mother, the day before his enlistment, is filled with concern for his family as well as hope and anticipation. In a letter to his sister Susanna on the same day, he is somewhat more direct:

New York April 18, 1861

Dear Susie,

You mustn't be made anxious or uneasy by what I am going to tell you. The President has called for 75,000 men, and the Seventh Regiment is ordered to Washington for its protection, with a great many men from Massachusetts and other States.

You mustn't think, dear Sue, that any of us are going to be killed; for they are collecting such a force there that an attack would be insane—that is, unless the Southerners can get their army up in an almost impossibly short space of time.

We go off to-morrow, and Father and Mother will be back three days after. [If] I could wait, I would; but if I don't go now, it is hardly probably I could go at all, and I know Mother wouldn't have me stay home at such a time. I can only write a few words now, but you shall hear from Washington.

By the morning of April 19, 1861, the streets surrounding the Seventh New York's armory, located at Third Avenue between East Sixth and Seventh Streets, were filled with carriages dropping off men at the building's drill hall. At 4:30 p.m., the men, with the band playing in the background, started marching down East Fourth Street. They reached Philadelphia later that night and were in the D.C./Baltimore area by April 23, 1861.

Philadelphia 9½ A.M. Saturday Apr 20/61

Dear Mother,

We have been here since two o'clock this morning & as soon as we hear that there is no trouble in Baltimore we shall go on. If there is a chance of our passage through Maryland being resisted we shall probably go by water.

Goodbye the drum is beating. I will write from Washington. Don't know what road we take yet.

***

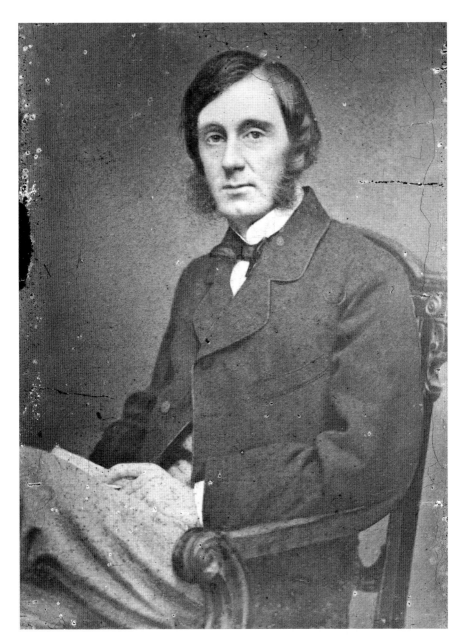

William Curtis. *Library of Congress, Washington, D.C.*

Annapolis Tuesday, April 23, 1861

Dear Father and Mother,

Last night at 6 o'clock we landed here, and have been quartered in the Naval School, where we are very comfortable indeed. The officers keep their plans to themselves, so we don't know how long we shall be here. They say the road to Washington is full of Secessionists, and the students have been in readiness for an attack for two or three days. I hope, unless the Colonel ascertains that the enemy is at Washington, as some think, that we shall start very soon. If they have possession of the city, of course, such a small force as ours could do no good outside of it. We have had no [news] *papers, so we know nothing of what is going on; but I, for one, do not believe the South Carolina army has got to the Capital quite yet. We didn't leave Philadelphia, until 2 p.m. on Saturday, and have had beautiful weather both on board the boat and since. If it had been rough when we were at sea, we should have had a fearful time, as we were piled together like pigs on the two upper decks and in the lower cabins, filling the boat perfectly full. When we arrived* [in Annapolis], *we found the Massachusetts men in a larger steam*[er] *run aground by the pilot, whom they immediately put in irons and wanted to kill. He is a Secessionist.*

General Butler, their commander, is an energetic, cursing and swearing old fellow. As soon as they got ashore, he sent a company into the town, took possession of the railroad depot, and set his men to work laying down the rails, which have been torn up by the Secessionists. He says "he'll be damned if he's going to be stopped by a lot of Maryland men." They had been trying to get off [the sandbar] *for three days. Our boat got them off at last....More than half their men were without water for two days, and had only two crackers per diem for some time, on board their boat.*

They [the Eighth Massachusetts] *are in all sorts of uniforms, and drill in the funniest way. All fishermen from Marblehead and shoemakers from Lynn, they seem itching for a fight.*

There are rumors that we start for to-morrow, and I think they have some foundation. The man who takes this letter is one of our company, who is afraid he won't be able to stand the march. I shall ask him to write on the outside of this whether anything new has turned up before he leaves. I shan't have a chance to see him to-morrow morning. If we go, it will be as early as 3 o'clock, a.m. The men are in good spirits; the stay here has freshened us all. Hope to see "Old Abe" soon.

On the morning of April 23, 1861, two messengers finally reached Annapolis from Washington. They were carrying a message from General Winfield Scott, ordering the Seventh New York and the Eighth Massachusetts to hurry to the capital. At that point, it was still in Union hands. The regiment prepared to depart along the damaged feeder rail line to Annapolis Junction, where the men expected to catch a train dispatched from Washington to bring them to the capital.

Washington, D.C. April 26, 1861, House of Representatives

Dearest Mother,

Just after closing my last [letter], at Annapolis, our Company got orders to fill their water-canteens, and be ready to receive three days' rations, as we were to start at 4 o'clock next morning [April 24].…We then found that Company 2 and Company 6 (ours) were to start for the Junction (Station between Baltimore and Washington) as advanced guard, and the others were to follow at about 9 a.m.

At the [Annapolis] depot we found the Massachusetts Company, which had taken possession. There was one old engine out [of] order, and half a dozen cars. One man had stepped up the night before, and said he could put it in order, because he had helped build it. It came from New England, of course. Another one jumped on when it was mended, got up the steam, and in a little while we were ready to start; so we packed our knapsacks into one car and started off in the other.

When we had gone about a mile by rail we had to get out, as the track was torn up in many places. We left our knapsacks on the train, which went back for the luggage of the rest of our men, while we trudged forward under a fearfully hot sun, with muskets loaded and cartridge-boxes full, ready for a brush at any moment. We had scout and skirmishers all around and about, for we had been positively assured that we should be attacked by a large body of cavalry.

We marched slowly along, pushing our howitzers on two baggage-cars, and stopping again and again to lay rails and make repairs on the roads. At length, about 2 o'clock, we came to a halt, and waited for the main body to come up, working meantime on a bridge which had been completely broken down, helped all the while by the Massachusetts boys, with whom we divided our rations, gaining thereby their enthusiastic admiration. Neither they nor we could have got through without each other's assistance. They are

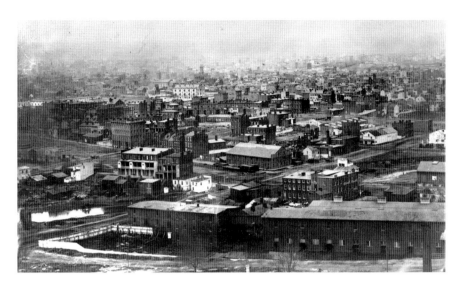

Early image of Washington, D.C. *Library of Congress, Washington, D.C.*

rough fellows, but of the best kind. The feeling of affection that has sprung up between us is really beautiful!

When the rest of our men had got up to where we stopped, and we had all rested and taken a nip at our crackers and beef, (six crackers and three pieces dried beef for three days!) we started off again, our two Companies still in advance as scouts; but we had to wait until after 6 o'clock, p.m., before the bridge was mended. In the meanwhile we had some very nice singing, patriotic songs being preferred, and at last got our howitzers over the bridge, and trudged along under a clear sky and splendid moon.

But 4 hours' sleep the night before, and 4 or 6 hours a night since we left New York, had not been sufficient to keep up our strength. However, we went on and on as before, stopping every half-hour and starting again, pushing and pulling on our old baggage-cars, sometimes up some very steep grades. Gradually, as time wore on, the men began to lie down every time we stopped, in larger and larger numbers, until at last everyone who was not at work was catching a sort of nap by the roadside. We had scouts out…so that we should have been warned in time of any enemy; but I don't believe it would have been possible to keep the men on their feet unless there had been an enemy really in sight. We actually fell asleep standing up, and scores of the men would drop their pieces and just catch themselves as they were toppling over.

We went through all sorts of defiles, where the Marylanders might have pounced upon us with great advantage, but though we had good evidence of their being about, from fresh tracks and newly torn-up rails, they took good care to keep well out of our way. The Annapolis men were perfectly certain we should be cut to pieces.

Before dawn, the men—sunburned, shivering in their damp uniforms and hungry—finally collapsed with fatigue, still wondering if the Maryland secessionists would ambush them and unaware that Annapolis Junction lay only two miles ahead.

At daybreak, 4½, we came to a halt about two miles from the Junction, perfectly overcome with sleep, shivering with cold, and good many of us grumbling in a quite a mutinous way. We built a dozen large fires—for the night air had gone through and through us, we had moved so slowly—and stood about them cogitating on the gloomy prospect before us. Provisions all gone—a good chance of having to march to Washington, twenty miles further, as we heard no train had come up to the Junction for us—and the expectation of being attacked in a little while, before we could get any rest. Our officers told us we should have to fight then, if ever.

While most men slept, advance scouts headed to Annapolis Junction where they soon learned that the Maryland militia, which had been clustered near the station, had suddenly departed the day before, and that a train sent from Washington that day in hopes of finding the New York men would return that morning. When the train arrived several hours later, the men were gathered at the station in wait, and they quickly ate the provisions that had been loaded into the cars in Washington.

Elizabeth Keckly, dedication of life. *Wikimedia Commons.*

The New York and Massachusetts troops could not both fit on the train, and the Massachusetts men wanted to stay back [and] avenge the attack on the Sixth Massachusetts regiment in Baltimore on April 18. When the train left at 9 a.m., it was filled with the Seventh New Yorkers, headed for their tumultuous welcome in Washington.

[W]e all turned out for a parade just as we were, covered with dust, and with our blankets slung over our shoulders....[We] marched straight up to the White House and through the grounds, where "old Abe" and family stood at the doors and saw us go by.

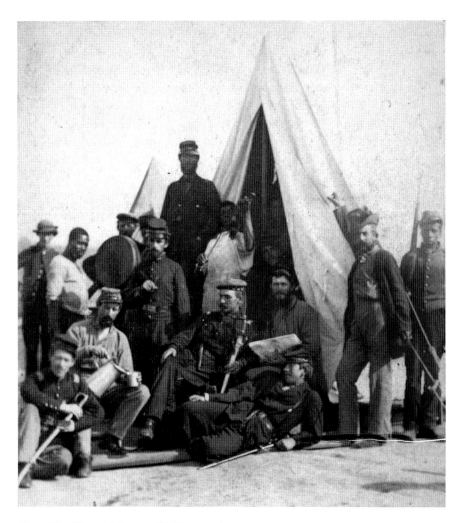

Camp life. *Library of Congress, Washington, D.C.*

*We then were distributed at different hotels in companies, and had our
first regular meal since we left New York.*

*That evening we marched up to the Capitol, and were quartered in the
House of Representatives, where we each have a desk, and easy-chair to
sleep in, but generally prefer the floor and our blankets, as the last eight days'
experience has accustomed us to hard beds. The Capitol is a magnificent
building, and the men all take the greatest pains not to harm anything Jeff
Davis shan't get it without trouble.*

95

[The Eighth Massachusetts] *arrived a day after us, and we all (being off duty) rushed out and cheered them; and they never let us go by now without clapping and hurrahing.*

When the Eighth Massachusetts men reached the Capitol on April 26, the First Pennsylvania, Sixth Massachusetts and Seventh New York volunteer regiments were already stationed there. The only remaining space for the newly arrived Massachusetts men was the Rotunda, open to the sky beneath the uncompleted dome.

Annie Haggerty and Robert Gould Shaw met in 1861. Annie was born in New York City on July 9, 1835, to Ogden and Elizabeth Haggerty. She and Shaw met at the opera in 1861 and stayed in touch during the war via letters.

To Shaw, the South was the aggressor, and if it took the end of slavery to redeem the honor of America, he was willing to fight for that.

In a February 1863 letter to Annie Haggerty, Shaw writes:

You know how many eminent men consider a Negro army of the greatest importance to our country at this time. If it turns out to be so, how fully repaid the pioneers in the movement will be, for what they may have to go through....I feel convinced I shall never regret having taken this step, as far as I myself am concerned; for while I was undecided I felt ashamed of myself, as if I were cowardly.

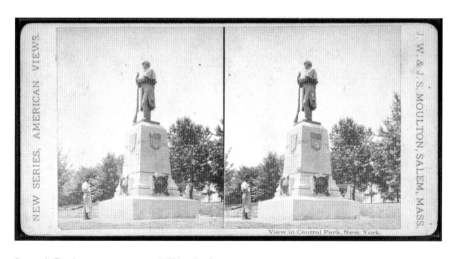

Seventh Regiment monument. *Wikimedia Commons.*

On April 17, 1863, Shaw became colonel of the Fifty-Fourth, and on May 2, 1863, Annie Haggerty and Robert Gould Shaw married in New York City.

By May 18, 1863, the Fifty-Fourth Regiment was at full capacity. Shaw and his men would face discrimination, hatred and bigotry the likes of which they may not have been fully prepared for. The psychological toll this took on the men under Shaw's command is important to recognize. Incidents of racism were pervasive. One such example was a Confederate Congress act:

Every white person being a commissioned officer, or acting as such, who, during the present war shall command Negroes or mulattoes in arms against the Confederate States, or who shall voluntarily aid Negroes or mulattoes in any military enterprise, attack or conflict in such service, shall be deemed as inciting servile insurrection, and shall if captured be put to death or be otherwise punished at the discretion of the court.

Through the summer of 1863, the regiment dealt with such injustices, preparing for the day they would be able to fight in a battle. Their time would happen with the Battle of Fort Wagner. The day before his death, in July 1863, the tenor of Shaw's writing changed dramatically. In a last letter to his wife, Annie, he spoke of his pride in his men. He spends a fair amount of time writing about casualties, injures and death. He also speaks of dirt and hunger.

There is hardly any water to be got here, and the sun and sand are dazzling and roasting us. I shouldn't like you to see me as I am now, I haven't washed my face since day before yesterday. My conscience is perfectly easy about it, though, for it was an impossibility, and everyone is in the same condition. Open air dirt, i.e. mud and is not like the indoor article....I have had nothing but crackers and coffee these two days. It seems like old times in the army of Potomac. Goodbye again, darling Annie.[169]

Shaw met with General Strong and learned that there would be a frontal assault on Fort Wagner that night. Before joining his men, Shaw located Edward L. Pierce, a correspondent for the *New York Daily Tribune*, and gave him some letters and personal items to pass on to Shaw's family in the event that he was killed in battle. The Shaw family, Annie included, issued a statement that they did not want Shaw's body moved. They requested that Shaw remain where he was—with his men. The attempt by the Confederates

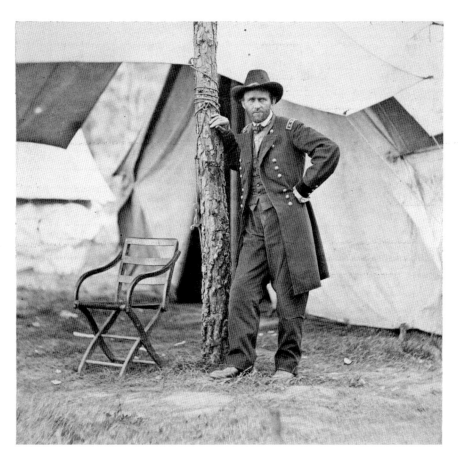

Ulysses S. Grant. *Library of Congress, Washington, D.C.*

to discredit the memory of the young colonel only served to solidify him as an icon. Poems and books would proclaim him and his men as the heroes that they were.

Reporter Edward Pierce recounted the hours leading up to the Fifty-Fourth's attack on Wagner. He spoke of the lack of rations and difficult trip they had to get to Wagner. The regiment left James Island on Thursday, July 16, at 9:00 p.m. and marched to Cole's Island. The men marched all night and the next day were left with only coffee and hardtack for sustenance. According to Pierce, "[T]hey breakfasted on the same fare, and had no other food before entering the assault on Fort Wagner in the evening....General Strong expressed a great desire to give them food and stimulants, but it was too late, as they were to lead the charge."[170] At approximately 7:00 pm, the

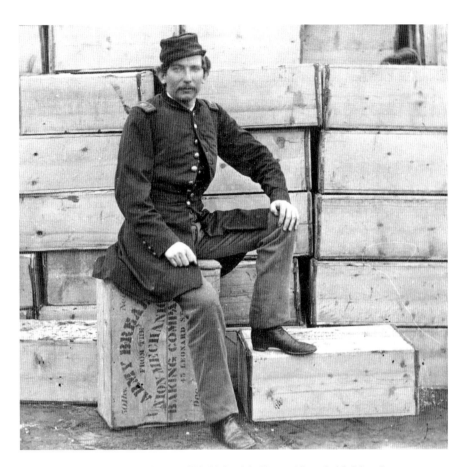

Picture of hardtack during the war. *U.S. National Archives and Records Administration.*

Fifty-Fourth was addressed by Colonel Shaw and General Strong, and then, at approximately 8:00 p.m. on July 18, 1863, the order was given for the Fifty-Fourth Massachusetts Infantry to charge Fort Wagner. The regiment advanced, first in quick time, then in double quick time. When Shaw reached the parapet, he was reported to have yelled "Onward boys" before being killed. Pierce indicated that the last time he saw Shaw was between 6:00 and 7:00 p.m. that evening when Shaw gave him the private letters described earlier and papers to be delivered to Shaw's father. Pierce noted after the charge that the men grieved "greatly at the loss of Colonel a Shaw, who seems to have acquired a strong hold on their affections."[171]

Nevertheless, the assault proved to be a turning point for black soldiers, serving to dismiss any lingering skepticism about the combat readiness of

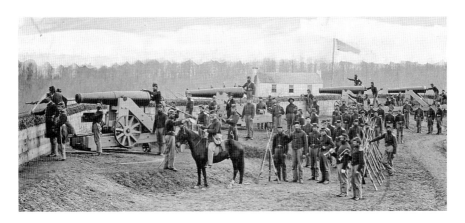

Fort Totten, D.C. *National Park Services.*

African Americans. General Ulysses S. Grant wrote to President Lincoln in August: "I have given the subject of arming the Negro my hearty support. They will make good soldiers and taking them from the enemy weakens him in the same proportion they strengthen us."

Regiments such as the Fifty-Fourth turned the tide of the war. President Lincoln understood the power of black soldiers fighting in the war:

> *You say you will not fight to free Negroes. Some of them seem to be willing to fight for you. When victory is won, there will be some black men who can remember that, with silent tongue and clenched teeth, and steady eye and well-poised bayonet, they have helped mankind on to this great consummation. I fear, however, that there will also be some white ones, unable to forget that with malignant heart and deceitful speech, they strove to hinder it.*

Annie Shaw was widowed at age twenty-eight when Colonel Shaw was killed at Fort Wagner on Morris Island, South Carolina. Shaw lived the remainder of her life as a widow, somehow content in knowing that she had been briefly married to the young colonel who gave his life for his country. She lived in France and Switzerland with her aging mother and her younger sister's family but eventually returned to the United States and kept up a sporadic correspondence with her sister-in-law, Josephine Shaw Lowell.

At middle age, Annie became ill and spent the last summer of her life in her old family home in Lenox. Annie Haggerty Shaw died on March 17,

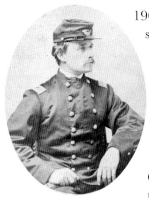

1907, at her sister's home in Boston at the age of seventy-one. She was buried in the Church on the Hill Cemetery in Lenox, Massachusetts, next to her mother, sister and brother-in-law.

Annie Haggerty Shaw died without ever seeing the Shaw Memorial on Boston Common. The bronze monument honors Colonel Robert Gould Shaw and the soldiers of the Fifty-Fourth Massachusetts Regiment. Sculptor Augustus Saint-Gaudens spent almost fourteen years completing the work.[172]

Robert Gould Shaw. *The New York Times.*

OPIATES, TRAUMA AND RECOVERY

The Union army had access to opium and morphine, and consumption of opium pills was widespread.[173] By the beginning of the Civil War, there was probably opium of some form in most household medicine cabinets.[174] "When called to the colors, whether Union or Confederate, doctors who used opiates liberally on civilian clients continued to use them liberally on their military patients."[175] Morphine was the preferred method of treating patients and wounded when syringes were in short supply; approximately thirty thousand units of morphine sulphate were dispensed to Union soldiers.[176] "Maimed and shattered survivors from a hundred battlefields, diseased and disabled soldiers released from hostile prisons, anguished and hopeless wives and mothers made so by the slaughter of those dearest to them, have found many of them temporary relief from their sufferings in opium."[177]

Opiates are a derivative of opium. Their use in pain management has a long history, as does the use of synthetic versions of the drug. "Opium is made by drying the milky resin that seeps from incisions made in unripe seedpods. An alternate method of harvesting morphine is to extract alkaloids from the mature dried plant stalks, to produce a fine brownish powder."[178] With respect to opium addition, according to Street:

> *The confirmed opium eater is habitually hopeless. His attempts at reformation have been repeated again and again; his failures have been as frequent as his attempts. He sees nothing before him but irremediable ruin.*

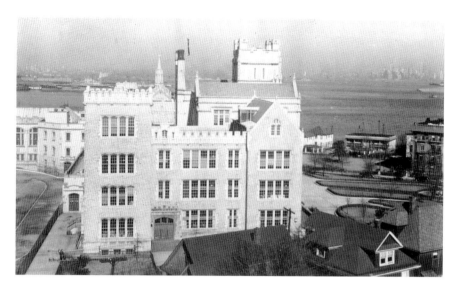

Curtis High School. *Wikimedia Commons.*

Under such circumstances of helpless depression, the following narratives from fellow-suffers and fellow-victims will appeal to whatever remains of his hopeful nature, with the assurance that others who have suffered even as he has suffered, and who have struggled as he has struggled, and have failed again and again as he has failed, have at length escaped the destruction which in his own case he has regarded as inevitable. The number of confirmed opium-eaters in the United States is large, not less, judging from the testimony of druggists in all parts of the country as well as from other sources, than eighty to a hundred thousand. The reader may ask who make up this unfortunate class and under what circumstances did they become enthralled by such a habit? Neither the business nor the laboring classes of the country contribute very largely to the number. Professional and literary men, persons suffering from protracted nervous disorders, women obliged by their necessities to work beyond their strength, prostitutes, and in brief all classes whose business or whose vices make special demands upon the nervous system, are those who for the most part compose the fraternity of opium eaters. The events of the last few years have unquestionably added greatly to their number. Maimed and shattered survivors from a hundred battlefields, disease and disabled soldiers released from hostile prisons, anguished and hopeless wives and mothers made so by the slaughter of those who were dearest to them, have found, many of them temporary relief from their sufferings in opium.[179]

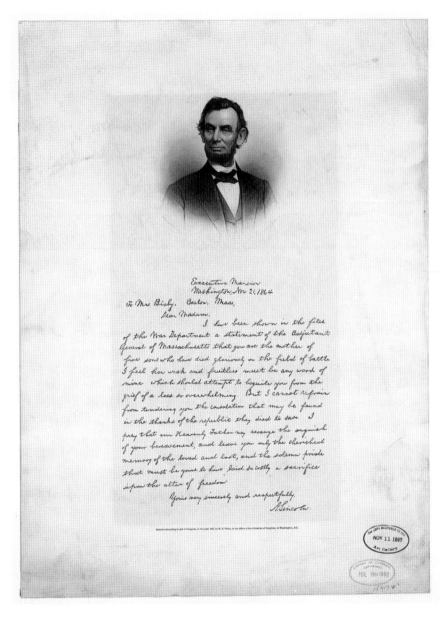

Letter between Abraham Lincoln and Mrs. Bixby. *Library of Congress, Washington, D.C.*

Additionally,

> *There are two temperaments in respect to this drug. With persons whom opium violently constricts or in whom it excites nausea, there is little danger that its use will degenerate into habit. Those however, over whose nerves it spreads only a delightful calm, whose feelings its tranquilizes, and in whom it produces a habitual state of reverie are those who should be upon their guard lest the drug to which in suffering they owe so much should become in time their direst of curse.*[180]

Apart from being used for a range of physical afflictions and as painkillers, opium and morphine were also issued to mitigate mental disorders caused by what we now know to be severe anxiety, flashbacks and recurrent traumatic images of war. Stress, fear and psychiatric breakdowns can be a byproduct of military conflict, and during the Civil War, opiates were used to treat symptoms such as numbness, madness, depression, insomnia, partial paralysis, gastrointestinal disorders, epilepsy, shortness of breath, chest pain and heart palpitations.

Secondary trauma also was an important factor during the war. While many of the letters contained in this book are from soldiers attempting to shield family members and loved ones from the horror of the war, this was not always so easy to accomplish, and those not physically present during a traumatic event could still be affected by the horrors witnessed directly by a brother, sister, husband or wife.[181]

The issue of psychological stress of the solider during the Civil War was not a huge issue for commanders due mainly to the fact that soldiers were expected to maintain a "manly" countenance, with very little tolerance for soldiers who did not. What were the options for soldiers unable to hide their psychological pain? Desertion, although this would have dire consequences if caught. A discharge of sorts, however, this might lead to charges of malingering and perpetuate the psychological pain of the soldier with very little relief in sight.[182] The ultimate penalty was execution.

> *Executions were intended both to eliminate, the contagion of weakness and to terrify the ranks into obedience. Such severe consequences must have discouraged many from seeking help. They certainly encouraged many others to resort to flight. Whether drafted or enlisted, though, the soldiers who fought for the North or for the South were certainly exposed [to] events that involved actual or threatened death or serious injury, or a threat to*

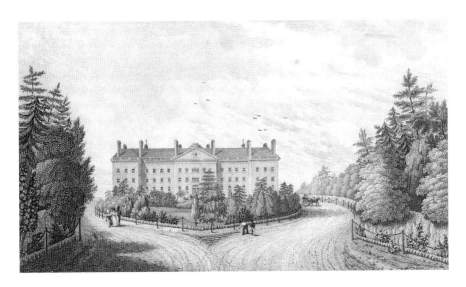

Bloomingdales Insane Asylum. *Wikimedia Commons.*

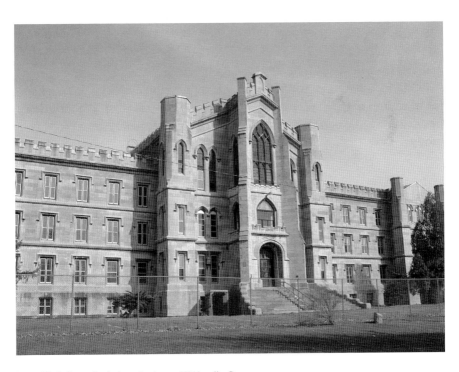

New York State Inebriate Asylum. *Wikimedia Commons.*

the physical integrity of self or others and there was adequate cause for a response that involved intense fear, helplessness and horror. It is impossible to know how many of the almost 400,000 deserters (about 10 percent of both armies) were running from personal demons, but it was the only resources short of execution or suicide available to those most acutely afflicted.[183]

As many writers have discussed, combat was not always the worst enemy the Civil War soldiers had to fear. "The common soldiers of the war faced each other only infrequently. Yet every day they risked their lives in battle with the unseen minions of corruption and decay, sometimes the results of their wounds, more often from the simple act of living through another day in camp."[184] According to poet and nurse Walt Whitman, "[F]uture years will never know the…hell and black infernal background, and it is best they should not."[185]

The following passage, from the book *My Life in the Irish Brigade*, the memoirs of Private William McCarter, captures much of what Walt Whitman is referencing:

Washington DC Wednesday morning December 17, 1862. The morning was clear and mild for the season. As we landed from the boat, the long lines of omnibuses and ambulances extending along the wharfs to convey our wounded soldiers to the various army hospitals in the city and suburbs were soon filled and started for their destination. Nine of my unfortunate comrades from various regiments and I were assigned to a large, old fashioned omnibus drawn by four horses. The coach started immediately. After a drive of about an hour along several streets of the Capital, and then into the country for a mile and a half, we arrived at the Eckington Army Hospital.…The nurse said encouragingly to me "We'll try and make a pretty good arm of it yet for you, leaving right afterwards," there were 50 beds in this building, 25 on either side, eleven of which were occupied on our arrival, but by eight pm the same night all of them were filled with wounded soldiers from the Battle of Fredericksburg. At two pm, I partook of the first good dinner since my departure from Philadelphia on the 1st of September. It consisted of plenty of baked chicken, buttered bread, hot coffee and mince pie. At eight am the patients were visited by the ward surgeon, Dr. Edling of New York, a gentleman in every sense of the term. He examined each man's wounds minutely, operating upon them if necessary, and left such directions with the nurses as the circumstances

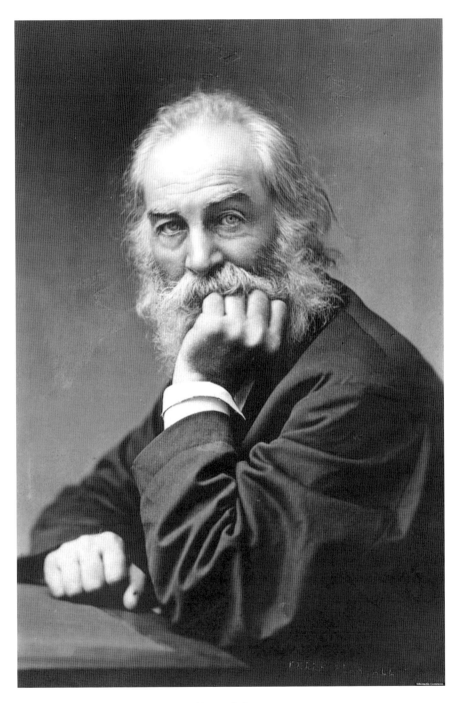

Walt Whitman. *Library of Congress, Washington, D.C.*

required. Visits were made by the ward surgeon, and young students, to the patients each morning at nine. We were also visited each evening at seven pm and sometimes during the day as cases demanded. These visits were often the occasion of considerable merriment, interest and curiosity, among the wounded soldiers. Often the surgeons themselves made a good joke or enjoyed a hearty laugh. For three weeks following the time, my wound in the right arm refused to heal and became more painful. It gradually grew worse, causing me constant uneasiness and suffering, almost depriving me of sleep. I rapidly lost my flesh and became as weak as a child. But strange to say my appetite, except on a few occasions, continued good. Dr. Edling said during one of his professional visits to me that it was the only favorable symptom in my case. I had been in this condition for perhaps 5 weeks when Dr. Edling entered our ward one morning on his visiting rounds. He seemed to take more than his usual interest in my case. He came right up to my bed upon which I was lying half dressed. The doctor seated himself beside me and took close, silent observations. Then rising, and moving away in a rather thoughtful and saddened manner, he left the ward without stopping to see any of the other patients. I did not know what to make of this but felt sure something was wrong. I passed an entirely sleepless night. My arm, which a few days before had commenced to swell near the shoulder, was now swollen to two times its natural size, assuming a most sickening and revolting appearance. I had not before thought the wound dangerous. But now, seeing my arm in such a condition and turning considerably scared—mortification and amputation to follow. Fear continually haunted my mind and racked me with pain, torturing my body. My physical appearance must have been wretched in the extreme. In twenty minutes, the doctor returned, accompanied by the head surgeon…and two students. They came up to my bed and seated themselves near one another on the unoccupied part of the bed. They asked me several questions concerning my feelings, appetite, and sleeping. Then after examining my wound very gently and passing a few private remarks among themselves in whispers (evidently not intended for my ears) they left me, as if not knowing what was best to be done in my case. I again laid down on my bed with no very agreeable thoughts. At one pm I partook of a hearty dinner brought me by nurse Zouvy consisting of rare roast beef, potatoes, bread, mince pie and a glass of bitter ale. Dr. Edling had ordered the latter for me. Nothing of note occurred til about 4pm. On the day following my introduction into my new quarters here, President Lincoln visited the Eckington Hospital, passing hurriedly from one ward to another. Upon entering my own apartment, he halted near

Copy of a letter from
Queen Victoria to
Mrs President Lincoln.

Osborne, April 1865

Though a stranger to you, I cannot remain silent when so terrible a calamity has fallen upon you and your country; and must personally express my deep and heartfelt sympathy with you under the shocking circumstances of your present dreadful misfortune. No one can better appreciate, than I can, who am myself utterly broken hearted by the loss of my own beloved husband, who was the light of my life, my stay, my all, – what your own sufferings must be; and I earnestly pray that you may be supported by Him, to whom alone the sorely stricken can look for comfort in their hour of heavy affliction. With the renewed expression of true sympathy, I remain, dear Madam, Your sincere friend, Victoria.

Letter between President Lincoln and Queen Victoria. *U.S. National Archives and Records Administration.*

the door and said in a quiet pleasing manner, "I can't stay boys. I hope you are all comfortable and getting along. I rly here. Goodbye." I have written about my life in the United States Army solely at the solicitation of my family and some of my friends. They wished to know about my experience as a soldier in the war for the Union. Owing to my unfortunate impediment in speaking, I had been prevented in the past from verbally relating my experiences, at least as fully as I would have liked. Thus I have resorted to my pen in the hope that the effort made will not only give the desired information in all respects, but will also provide satisfactory, amusing and perhaps in some degree instructive lessons about the war.[186]

Orphans were another product of the war. The 1860s saw the proliferation of orphanages, which catered not only to children who had lost both parents but also to those who were essentially refugees and those who had lost a father during the war either physically or mentally.

Even if fathers walk through the door following their time in service, it did not mean that they were fully back. Post-traumatic stress disorder is a modern term for a disorder as old as fighting and war itself. Certainly some of the Civil War soldiers returning home must have suffered in varying degrees from some form of it....[C]hildren had been dealing with the trauma of the war from the beginning. Now, likely, they expected everything to return to the way it had been before. As fathers, and other loved ones returned home it must have been a huge strain on the children to see how the war had changed them. A depressed and alcohol dependent man may have replaced the once kind and loving father. Who was this man? What happened to daddy?[187]

James Henry Gooding of the Fifty-Fourth Massachusetts was a product of the Colored Orphan Asylum. According to historian Ray Anthony Shepard, Gooding was bought out of slavery and taken to New York City's Colored Orphan Asylum. He was taken care of by Quakers and learned to read and write at the orphanage.[188] Sadly, this orphanage burned down in the New York Draft Riots of 1863; however, other resources would be born out of the ashes of war. The New England Home for Little Wanderers was founded in 1865 by ten Boston businessmen. The goal was to care for children left homeless and/or orphaned by the Civil War. It was not the intention that it would become a permanent home for the children. Many

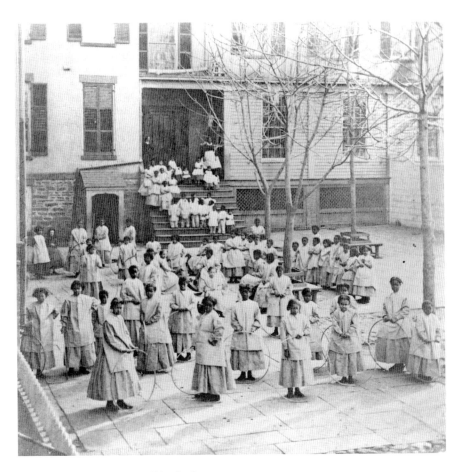

Colored Orphan Asylum. *Wikimedia Commons.*

of the children ended up living new lives with families in other parts of the country and were transported to their new homes by trains in what became known as the Orphan Train Movement.[189] Thousands of orphans left cities such as New York for lives with new families throughout the country. Charles Loring Brace, the founder of the Children's Aid Society, was a large driver behind this movement. He started with the newsboys who sold papers in the streets of cities like New York. In the post–Civil War period, he placed thousands of children with new families. His dear friend Elizabeth Schuyler, upon his death, spoke of his ability to find creative solutions for the homeless children of New York City.[190]

According to writer Gene Fynes, in his article "Orphanage for Children of Iowa Civil War Soldiers Opened 150 Years Ago on November 16," Civil

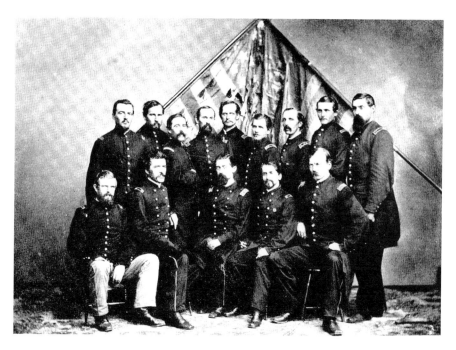

Forty-Fourth New York Regiment. *Emory University.*

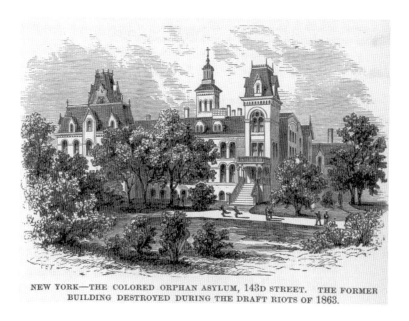

NEW YORK—THE COLORED ORPHAN ASYLUM, 143D STREET. THE FORMER BUILDING DESTROYED DURING THE DRAFT RIOTS OF 1863.

Colored Orphan Asylum. *Wikimedia Commons.*

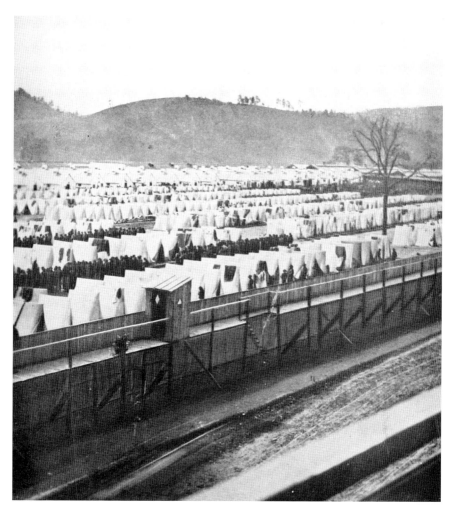

Elmira Prison. *Library of Congress, Washington, D.C.*

War orphans were indeed a "casualty" of the war. These were children who either had two parents who died or were unable to care for them. Fynes writes about how fathers either died or were too emotionally or physically disabled to care for their children and mothers often breaking under the strain of being home alone for the entirety of the war or dying themselves.[191]

NEW YORK AND D.C. HOSPITAL FACILITIES CARING FOR CIVIL WAR VETERANS

T he war saw an influx of either new hospitals or changes to existing hospitals. In 1855, Congress established the Government Hospital for the Insane, later St. Elizabeth's Hospital. The purpose of the hospital was to provide "the most humane care and enlightened curative treatment of the insane of the army and navy of the United States, and of the District of Columbia." The belief was that by distracting patients, the awful memories would be replaced. Distractions included church services, educational lectures, books and musical instruments, including several pianos. Caregivers attempted "to render the institution not only a good hospital, but a kind and sympathizing home."[192] The notion that care, empathy and medicine should work together found its way to other cities.

Healing and caregiving, as we have seen throughout the book, comes in many forms and through many people. Dr. Susan McKinney, as stated earlier, was the first African American female physician in New York State and the third in the nation, and she graduated from New York Medical College for Women in 1870 with the highest grade in the class. When that institution closed in 1918, students transferred to New York Medical College. Thus, New York Medical College claims to be among the first medical schools to admit women. Expansion of the college's facilities and programs began early in its history. By 1872, the medical staff had moved into larger quarters made available by the New York Ophthalmic Hospital at Third Avenue and Twenty-Third Street. This institution, one of only two in New York City at the time for the treatment of ophthalmic diseases, had been placed

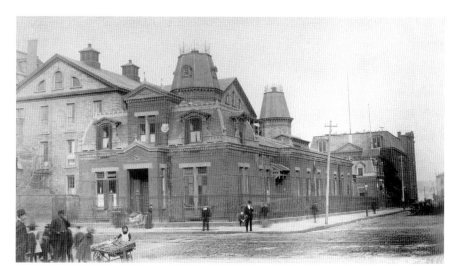

Bellevue Hospital. *Wikimedia Commons.*

under the college's supervision in 1867. Students were thus able to enroll in graduate study in ophthalmology and had the opportunity to earn another degree. In 1875, Metropolitan Hospital opened as a municipal facility on Ward's Island, staffed largely by the faculty of New York Medical College. The relationship, which continues, is among the nation's oldest continuing affiliations between a private medical school and a public hospital.

Faculty began to consider the desirability of establishing a hospital connected to the school to afford closer opportunities for clinical instruction. The Flower Free Surgical Hospital, built by New York Medical College in 1889, was the first teaching hospital in the country to be owned by a medical college. It was constructed at York Avenue and Sixty-Third Street with funds given largely by Congressman Roswell P. Flower, later governor of New York. It became possible now, for the college "to embrace under its jurisdiction a free hospital for treatment of the poor and for clinical instruction of its students" as the minutes of the board of trustees duly recorded. New York Medical College owes its founding in 1860 to the vision of a group of civic leaders in New York City who believed that medicine should be practiced with greater sensitivity to the patients. The group, led by William Cullen Bryant, was particularly concerned with the condition of hospitals and medical education. Bryant was zealously devoted to the branch of medicine known as homeopathy, which, among its tenets, advocated moderation in medicinal dosage, exercise, a good diet, fresh air and rest in treating illness.

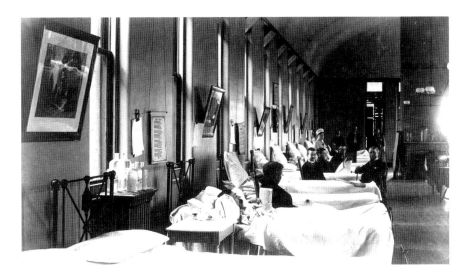

Bellevue Hospital. *Wikimedia Commons.*

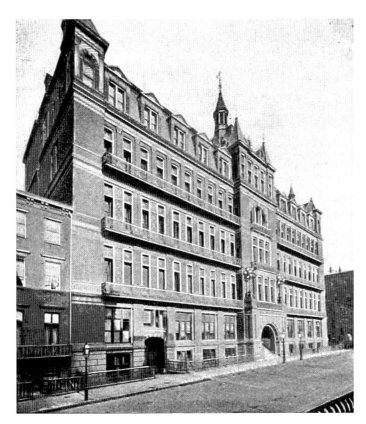

New York Hospital at West Fifteenth Street near Fifth Avenue. *The British Library.*

Recreation therapy in modern times is well integrated in overall holistic healthcare programs for patients. Recreational therapy involves utilizing a variety of activities in order to help the physical, emotional and social functions of patients and enhance their abilities to live productive lives. After the Civil War, recreational therapy at places like the Bath VA Hospital were inconsistent at best in the late 1880s.

> *Since the middle of the 19th Century, the federal government has recognized the need to provide care for some American veterans beyond the monetary support of pension benefits. Most people are familiar with the system of national homes for disabled Union Veterans that opened around the country after the Civil War, but Congress established one of the first national homes for Regular Army and volunteer soldiers a generation on earlier. Known initially as the Military Asylum in Washington, D.C. And later as the U.S. soldiers' Home—made famous during the Civil War as the site of President Abraham Lincoln's summer retreat—the institution offered the first official sanctuary for the relief and support of invalid, disabled, and homeless veterans.*[193]

Most soldiers who entered the soldiers' home suffered from a host of physical and psychological illnesses directly related to their military service. According to the register of patients admitted to the hospital from 1872 to 1927, some ailments the patients suffered from included: alcoholism, diarrhea, tuberculosis, conjunctivitis, paralysis, asthma, hernias and common sprains.[194] In New York City, public and private hospitals have been essential to the care of New Yorkers, with public hospitals accepting all who needed care.[195]

Bellevue opened in 1736 as New York City's Almshouse. New York provided cash allowances to assist poorer individuals with their healthcare issues. Individuals utilizing the city's Almshouse tended to be older, orphans, individuals with mental health issues or the very sick. Places like the city's Almshouse were a source of refuge for many.[196]

The rapid rise in the reported number of hospitals from 178 in 1872 to more than 4,000 in 1910 stemmed only in part from the growth of hospitalization. After all, more hospital beds might have been accommodated in fewer institutions by increasing their average size. Mental hospitals in America developed in this way, increasing their capacity rather than feverishly multiplying in number.[197]

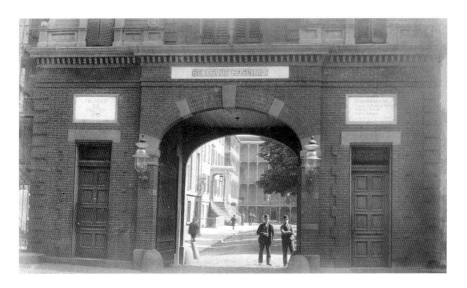

Bellevue Hospital. *Wikimedia Commons.*

The Floating Hospital started in October 1866 as charitable trips by steamboat entrepreneur John Sarin for the benefit of newsboys, war veterans and those in need. The first floating hospital ship was the *Emma Abbott*, named after the singer. Abbott was an early supporter of the Floating Hospital and was crucial to its success.[198] In July 1873, *New York Times* editor George F. Williams was crossing the City Hall Park when he saw five children under a tree. One of the children stated they were playing as though they were in the country. Williams told the story to another editor, and together they wrote the editorial "Why Cannot the Poor Children Go to the Country in the Hot Weather?" It was out of this article that the "Fresh Air Work" started. Williams's first step was excursions for newsboys and other underserved youth. After one of these trips, a small boy approached Williams and asked what was to become of sick children on these trips. It was through this that the Floating Hospital was born. By 1903, there were two Floating Hospitals in New York: the *Emma Abbott* and the *Helen C. Julliard*, which accommodated three thousand mothers and infants daily. One hospital was on either side of New York City, and each was equipped for hundreds of sick, impoverished residents of the city. The hospitals operated from early July until late September.

As time went on, the hospital had three landings daily on each side of the city and in Brooklyn. The first was at 8:00 a.m. The hospital approached the pier with hundreds of mothers carrying the sick children who waited for the approach of the hospital. The mothers presented a ticket containing the name, address, age and diagnosis signed by a physician. Thousands of mothers and children were cared for over the years.

The Civil War saw an unprecedented influx of veterans. While many families of soldiers believed they would be able to care for these returning veterans at home, many quickly learned what a daunting task this was from a physical, financial and emotional standpoint.[199] In 1866, the National Asylum for Disabled Volunteer Soldiers was created by Congress. In 1872, New York State passed an act to create a New York Soldiers Home. Bath, New York, was selected for several reasons, including the fact that the community had raised $23,000 toward building a home and the area had the environment for a good sewage system.[200] In 1878, the New York State Soldiers and Sailors Home (NYSSSH) saw construction of three buildings. Between 1878 and 1900, several other buildings were erected, including a 150-bed hospital, a farmhouse, a house for the chaplain, two additional hospital wards and new barracks.[201]

By the late 1800s, the hospital was up and running, and by 1902, it was able to report on the operations and functioning as well as overall care. An annual report from the Bath VA facility listed causes of death in 1902–3. The leading causes of death included heart disease; brain diseases such as stroke, cerebral syphilis and cerebral hemorrhage; pulmonary disease such as pulmonary pneumonia and TB; and cancer.[202]

Interestingly, there were twenty-two deaths with no cause listed. Rather, the place of death was listed: 50 percent of these deaths were "on furlough"; 28 percent "soon after reaching hospital"; 10 percent in barracks; 2 percent "in boiler house"; and 10 percent killed by locomotive. According to the Bath VA Medical Center 125th Anniversary Booklet, previous years also saw deaths that included suicides, drownings and falls. These deaths imply a possible mental health component. The Bath VA also experienced issues related to residents' alcoholism. According to General Order no. 324 (September 18, 1886):

> *The Superintendent again calls attention to the fact that the permission to leave the grounds on Sunday, is for the purpose of attending Divine Services, and that only. He regrets however, to know that many take advantage of the privilege to frequent the Rum Holes in our vicinity and the town. As a general thing, services of the churches are over in time to enable those attending to return by 12:30 and it is made the duty of the police at the bridge to report all*

who cross the bridge after that hour, and any man so reported will be deprived of the privilege of going out on Sunday for six months, and if this does not have the desired effect more summary measures will be resorted to. This order will be read at dinner and supper and at the 1ˢᵗ and 2ⁿᵈ tables so that no man can plead as an excuse that he did not hear it.[203]

Rules of Admission for the NYSSSH (Bath VA) from 1880 to 1916

- Been honorably discharged
- Been born in or been a resident of NYS for one year preceding admission
- Been disabled from a wound or wounded while in service of the United States
- No property or means of support
- No relatives of sufficient ability to maintain him and if he had to deposit the whole amount received with the treasurer of the Home
- Not been an "inmate" of another national home or discharged from one within the last three months[204]

Discharges from the Bath VA became less complicated as time went on. According to General Order no. 188 from the fall of 1884, "The following named inmate is hereby discharged upon his own application and statement that he is able to maintain himself. He will be readmitted only by an order from the Board of Trustees and upon such conditions as they may impose."

In the early 1880s, according to hospital General Order no. 202, "John A. Smith, late co. K, 13ᵗʰ New York Infantry Vol. was absent from the hospital long enough to be discharged from the hospital. He would only be allowed to be readmitted upon written application and permission." The Bath VA was originally supposed to be a stopgap for veterans with fairly minor medical issues. As the soldiers aged, their needs evolved.[205] By 1917, discharge could be completed "upon his application therefore, unless he be at the time under charges for misconduct."[206]

From 1861 through 1865, general hospitals treated more than one million soldiers. They had a mortality rate of 8 percent. Washington's sixteen General Hospitals had nearly thirty thousand beds.

In 1852, financier William Wilson Corcoran purchased 191 acres to use as a country estate in Washington, D.C. In 1862, Harewood Hospital was built on Corcoran's property in a "V" pavilion style. It operated between September 1862 and May 1866, caring for wounded soldiers. Harewood consisted of frame buildings and tents. The hospital had nine wards, with 63 beds each, for a total of 945 beds. Hospital tents with 6 beds each were added. At one point, 312 hospital tents were in use on the site, with a capacity of 1,872 beds. In December 1864, the hospital had 2,080 beds. It was the last of Washington's Civil War hospitals to close.

JUDICIARY SQUARE GENERAL HOSPITAL

Between 1861 and 1862, the U.S. Sanitary Commission urged the government to build pavilion-style hospitals, instead of renting buildings ill-adapted for hospitals. As a result, Armory Square, Mount Pleasant and Judiciary Square Hospitals were completed in 1862. These state-of-the-art hospitals featured separate wards, or pavilions, radiating from a central corridor. They were based on the British design first used in the Crimean War and emphasized ample ventilation.

Sisters of Mercy took over operation of the Washington Infirmary in 1855. When the Civil War began in 1861, they offered the infirmary to the government. When it burned down later that year, the government seized the private mansions of Senator Stephen A. Douglas of Illinois, Vice President John C. Breckinridge of Kentucky and Senator Henry Rice of Minnesota. These dwellings became the Douglas General Hospital.

The War Department asked the Sisters to take charge of Douglas Hospital on December 23, 1861. Former superior at the infirmary Sister Mary Colette O'Connor served as superintendent. She possessed remarkable executive abilities and a tender heart. Unfortunately, her health was weakened by the grueling work, and Sister Mary Colette died on July 16, 1864.

The Sisters of Mercy compassionately cared for the sick at Douglas and prepared the dying for eternity. More than six hundred Catholic sisters served during the Civil War, and one hundred of these were Sisters of Mercy. The only organized, experienced and available nurses in the country, they nursed the wounded; organized housekeeping, cooking and distributing food; and provided laundry services. They often risked death by tending to patients with contagious diseases. The large pavilion-style hospitals

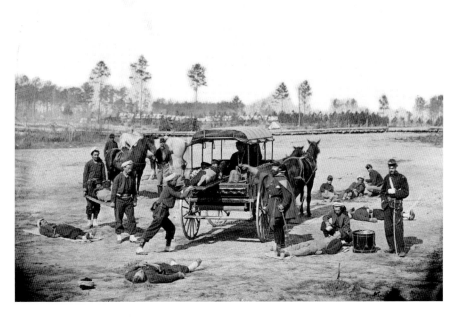

Civil War ambulance. *Library of Congress, Washington, D.C.*

constructed during the war comprised one hundred or more independent wooden barracks that were well ventilated and could be easily isolated in case of disease outbreak or fire. The hospitals bought food locally and grew vegetables in gardens at the facilities. Ample supplies of fresh water and herds of dairy cows contributed to the welfare of the patients; some hospitals had their own icehouses and breweries.

An important part of recovery for many patients was being in a healthy environment. According to journalist Noah Brooks:

> *All Washington* [is] *a great hospital for the wounded in the great battle now going forward in Virginia. Boatloads of unfortunate and maimed men are continually arriving at the wharves and are transported to the various hospitals in and around Washington in ambulances or upon stretchers, some of the more severely wounded being unable to bear the jolting of the ambulances....There are twenty-one hospitals in this city and vicinity and every one of them is full of the wounded and the dying.*

The buildings at Florida Avenue and Sixth Street were converted into Campbell Hospital to care for the wounded. They served primarily as

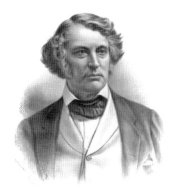

Charles Sumner. *Library of Congress, Washington, D.C.*

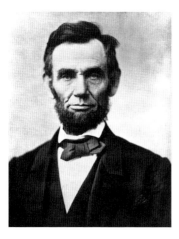

Abraham Lincoln. *Library of Congress, Washington, D.C.*

wards, but the center building housed a dining room and kitchen. There were eleven structures total with six hundred beds. The Medical Department installed ventilation, and louvered exits were used in winter with inlets near the stoves. Converted hospitals had many logistical issues. For example, some converted barracks hospitals were not connected to the municipal water supply, thus making distributing water and removing waste challenging. Transporting the wounded from battlefields to converted hospitals was also challenging. Wounded soldiers were transported in rickety two-wheeled vehicles—of course, assuming the wounded were actually removed from the battlefield, which was not always the case. Ambulances were introduced during the war, and in March 1864, Congress created an ambulance corps for all Union armies.

Walt Whitman spent a fair amount of time caring for the wounded at barracks-style hospitals, like Campbell and Carver, which he called, "a wall'd and military city regularly laid out, and guarded by squads of sentries."

The Washington, D.C. military hospitals such as Harewood, Carver and Mount Pleasant were located on the periphery of the city, near President Lincoln's summer cottage at the Soldiers' Home. Both President and Mrs. Lincoln frequently visited these hospitals in order to provide comfort to the soldiers. The president passed Harewood Hospital on his commute between his summer retreat and the White House, and he sometimes stopped there for a visit. According to this excerpt from *Lincoln's Men* by William Davis, President Lincoln enjoyed visiting soldiers in military hospitals:

> *Unannounced, he might simply appear in a ward to talk with the men in their cots. "I can't stay, boys," he said in one hospital where he rapidly*

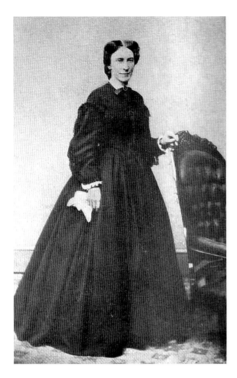

Amanda Akin. *Smithsonian Institute.*

went from ward to ward. "I hope you are all comfortable and getting along nicely here." When time allowed, he went to each bed, shaking hands with every soldier in turn. What he saw often left him shocked and horrified. His friend and companion [Ward Hill Lamon] *sometimes saw the president disturbed "almost beyond his capacity to control either his judgment or his feelings."*[207]

LETTERS AND APPEALS FROM MOTHERS TO PRESIDENT LINCOLN

"I am a colored woman and my son was strong and able to fight for his country and the colored people have as much to fight for as any," declared Hannah Johnson from Buffalo, York, in a July 31, 1863 letter to President Abraham Lincoln.

Johnson's son was a soldier in the Fifty-Fourth Massachusetts Infantry of the United States Colored Troops. Knowing that her son might die in battle, Johnson was deeply concerned that he, and thousands of other

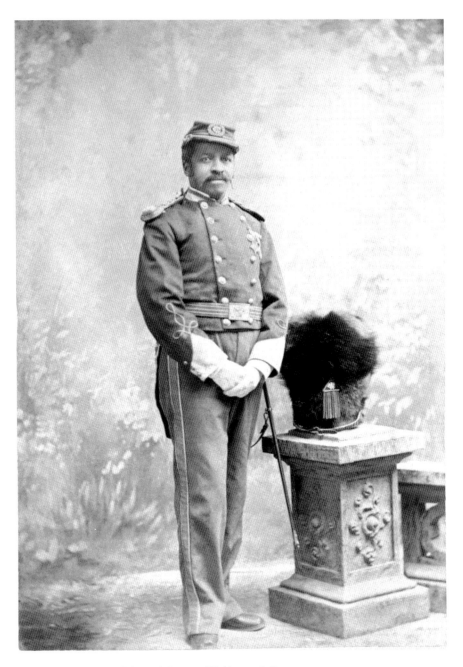

Christian Fleetwood. *Library of Congress, Washington, D.C.*

black soldiers, would be treated poorly despite their service. In her letter to President Lincoln, Johnson claims the right of personal petition to the highest official in the land, despite that, as an African American woman, her status as a citizen was not clear. The letter offers a glimpse of the way African Americans viewed the war, their place in it and their relationship to Lincoln.

Close to 180,000 black men served in the Union army by war's end. Most of them were slaves who had fled from the Confederate states. Three-fourths of all Northern black men volunteered. They were segregated in units initially led by white officers and were often assigned the most arduous jobs and the most dangerous combat roles. To add insult to injury, they were denied equal pay. This imposed a double burden to fight against enemy forces and to protest against the "friendly fire" of racial prejudice. These inequities kept at least some men from joining the army, but more often than not, they eagerly enrolled with a strong commitment to serve their country and rescue their people from bondage. But there were other unique obstacles in their way, which Johnson turned to the president to address. She made clear to Lincoln that she had weighed the pros and cons of her son's enlistment beforehand. She even considered the horror that he might be taken prisoner. Confederates identified black soldiers as slave insurrectionists, regardless of their antebellum status. They released their wrath on captives in the form of summary executions and re-enslavement, as if they had engaged in high treason against the Southern nation-state. This was a clear violation of the Lieber Code of conduct in war, which mandated humane treatment of prisoners of war regardless of race.

Johnson initially felt certain that Lincoln "will never let them sell our colored soldiers for slaves, if they do he will g[et] them back quck[.] He will retallyate and stop it." Her own son survived the assault on Fort Wagner and was not captured, but many others weren't so lucky. Yet the president and other officials did not respond swiftly enough to protect them. If black soldiers suffered equal risks of losing their lives, Johnson asked the president, "So why should not our enemies be compelled to treat him the same, Made to do it."

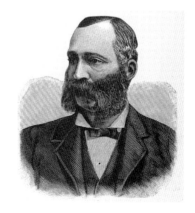

Charles Purvis. *National Library of Medicine.*

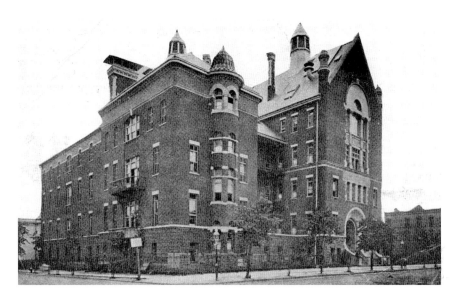

German Hospital. *Wikimedia Commons.*

With respect to the Confederate soldiers, Johnson argued that "they have lived in idleness all their lives on stolen labor and made savages of the colored people, but they now are so furious because they are proving themselves to be men." Additionally, "[Y]ou must put the rebels to work in State prisons to making shoes and things, if they sell our colored soldiers, till they let them all go. And give their wounded the same treatment, it would seem cruel, but their [is] no other way."

She also called forth a long tradition of African American struggles against unjust laws that had buttressed the entire edifice of slavery. "Ought one man to own another, law for or not, who made the law, surely the poor slave did not, so it is wicked, and a horrible Outrage, there is no sense in it," she stated and queried, all at once. Crimes against humanity over centuries could not be justified or made right by the perverse logic of slaveholders who were self-styled victims of their own creation. It is important to remember that for all the trials that black soldiers faced, they gained much. The mere sight of black men in blue uniforms was a powerful statement whose meaning was not lost on Confederate soldiers. Black men who took up arms against former masters proved their valor on the battlefield. Their sense of dignity and self-respect were palpable. They were rewarded with gratitude and everlasting respect in the eyes of their families, communities and in the nation at large.

In the process, a new path to citizenship was opened—but one that only men could achieve. So what about women like Hannah Johnson, and those who lived in the direct line of fire in the South? By what route could they advance their standing?

Johnson's letter demonstrates that women like her were increasingly leading themselves, their children and other family members out of slavery as men's enlistment accelerated. They fled to contraband camps or set up makeshift shantytowns close to Federal lines when they were not welcomed within them. Additional concerns included hostility from Union soldiers upon fleeing to Union lines. Women were also disproportionately represented among slaves left behind on the homefront still forced into plantation labor. Those who were related to soldiers and could not be rescued by them were especially vulnerable to reprisal.

When Martha Glover's husband escaped to join the army, she was left to deal with the consequence. "I have had nothing but trouble sin[c]e you left," she wrote him. "They abuse me because you went & say that they will not take care of our children & do nothing but quarrel with me all the time and beat me scandalously." Her husband's departure was bittersweet no matter how noble the cause: "You ought not to left me in the fix I am in & all these little helpless children to take care of." She wished he had waited until she could follow him: "for I do nothing but grieve all the time about you."

Many other women found ways of contributing to the war effort wherever they were. Susie King Taylor, a fugitive slave, served as cook, nurse, teacher and laundress for a South Carolina regiment. "There were 'loyal women' as well as men, in those days, who did not fear shell or shot, who cared for the sick and dying: women who camped and fared as the boys did," she recalls in her postwar memoir. "They were hundreds of them who assisted the Union soldiers by hiding them and helping them to escape. Many were punished for taking food to prison stockades for the prisoners."

Taylor informs her readers that "many lives were lost—not men alone but noble women as well." And yet she knew that their nobility was often denied and ignored. She insisted that the memory of black women's wartime deeds be preserved: "These things should be kept in history before the people." Black women were often perceived to be nuisances, beggars and thorns in the side of their allies, far afield from the respect heralded in verse and song for white Union and Confederate women.

Lucy Chase, a white volunteer at a contraband camp in Virginia, noted the arrival of women and children with fathers and "husbands [who] are with the army, they know not where.…[T]hey are alone, with no one to comfort them," and yet they claimed their own contributions and sacrifices, as though they too had "entered the army."

In the summer of 1818, when Abraham Lincoln was nine years old, his mother, Nancy, caught the "milk-sick," a then mysterious disease caused by drinking the milk of cows that had eaten white snakeroot (brucellosis). Within a week, she was dead. In adulthood, Lincoln confided to a friend about how lonely he felt in the months afterward, and how he found solace in the Bible stories his mother had told him; the words restored her voice to his mind's ear. "All that I am, or hope to be," he said, "I owe to my angel mother." It is therefore interesting to hear of the story of Hannah Johnson as well as to see the letters Lincoln received from mothers regarding the war. These letters are filled with pain, trauma and anger. But ultimately, they are also filled with healing.

Possibly Lincoln thought of his mother, Nancy Lincoln, when he received letters from women whose sons were fighting in the Civil War. Here follow samples of correspondence between Lincoln and Civil War mothers. As stated earlier in the book, trauma during wartime extends to family members. Some of the more salient examples of trauma and the war come from the writings of mothers to President Lincoln. Letters have been edited for length but retain their original spelling and grammar.

***

President U States
Hon. A Lincoln

Dear Sir

Will you excuse my daring to address you, and enclosing this petition for my eldest son, for, your kind consideration. It will tell you all I need, and allow me to say a few words. I know you will listen to them for you have a kind heart, and my story is a sad one. I am a widow left with only these two sons, who have both left me, to fight for the good cause and I am proud to send them forth although they leave me desolate, and, heartbroken, as they were all I had, for my support, and were my only hope in this world, but I have given them up, but trust in God's mercy, to return them to me, some day. My eldest son is First Lieut in the 15th Regiment, and educated for the army wishes a permanent place in it my youngest son, is a Private soldier in Gen Duryea' 5th Regiment Advance Guards, now at Fort Monroe. He is a druggist by Profession and almost a Physician. He was my only stay, because the youngest and to have him perhaps forever taken away from me almost kills me. My health is extremely delicate and if he could only have a higher place than a private in the Regiment, would make me feel better if he could assist in the Medical Staff in the Hospital, perhaps I am wild to ask such things but I know you can do all things.... Dont dear Mr Lincoln refuse to listen to a Widowed Mother prayer. Will you look favorable on this petition? Let me ask your forgiveness for trespassing but you will excuse a broken hearted woman.

Cornelia Ludlow Beekman
July 1861

***

To: The Hon. Pres. A Lincoln

I humbly pray you to pardon my son Benjamin F Stevens who is under arrest & probably sentenced for going to sleep on guard in the 49th regt Indiana Vols....He is but sixteen years of age. I humbly ever pray

Mrs. Eliza J Stevens
Seymour, Indiana
April 1862

***

Excellent Sir

My good friend says I must write to you and she will send it. My son went in the 54th [Massachusetts] regiment. I am a colored woman and my son was strong and able as any to fight for his country and the colored people have as much to fight for as any. My father was a Slave and escaped from Louisiana before I was born morn forty years agone I have but poor education but I never went to schol, but I know just as well as any what is right between man and man. Now I know it is right that a colored man should go and fight for his country, and so ought to a white man. I know that a colored man ought to run no greater risques than a white, his pay is no greater his obligation to fight is the same. So why should not our enemies be compelled to treat him the same, Made to do it.

My son fought at Fort Wagoner but thank God he was not taken prisoner, as many were I thought of this thing before I let my boy go but then they said Mr. Lincoln will never let them sell our colored soldiers for slaves, if they do he will get them back quck he will retallyate and stop it. Now Mr Lincoln dont you think you oght to stop this thing and make them do the same by the colored men they have lived in idleness all their lives on stolen labor and made savages of the colored people, but they now are so furious because they are proving themselves to be men, such as have come away and got some education. It must not be so. You must put the rebels to work in State prisons to making shoes and things, if they sell our colored soldiers, till they let them all go. And give their wounded the same treatment. it would seem cruel, but their no other way, and a just man must do hard things sometimes, that shew him to be a great man. They tell me some do you will take back the [Emancipation] Proclamation, don't do it. When you are dead and in Heaven, in a thousand years that action of yours will make the Angels sing your praises I know it…

Will you see that the colored men fighting now, are fairly treated. You ought to do this, and do it at once, Not let the thing run along meet it quickly and manfully, and stop this, mean cowardly cruelty. We poor oppressed ones, appeal to you, and ask fair play. Yours for Christs sake

Hannah Johnson
Buffalo, New York
July 1863

***

Sir,
I have as you know, a son, an only and most dearly loved son, in the Southern Army; and I know, am well assured that if I can reach Richmond I shall be enabled to procure for him an honorable discharge from the army and an opportunity of being once more united (in a foreign land) to his

mother and child. I ask you now for the permit to go south, and oh—Mr Lincoln by the love you bear to your dear ones who are yet spared to you, as well as that you bear for those, that whom God has called to await you in another and a happier world, grant my petition. Let me go, and if I should fail in the main object of my journey—still I shall once more see my child face to face, and his little boy, may take away a memory of his father, which otherwise he may never have.

You may trust my honor, for taking nothing contraband, nor compromising my government by letter or word of mouth—Yield to my entreaties and receive the ever grateful remembrance of

Yours Respectfully

Harriette B. Prentice
Louisville, Kentucky
January 1864

***

dear Sir!

Permit me the honor of an interview, with your excellency. I have ventured again alone my Husband's official duties debar him from accompanying me. Though my errand in behalf of my Son in-law Capt. John D. O'Connell of the Regular Army—necessitates immediate attention—The Captain's situation likewise compels his constant presence, where he is in comd. over the Recruiting Service of the 14th Infty at Fort Trumbull New London, Conn. and where he has himself been recruiting his own health, from serious wounds, and I am most happy to inform your Excellency, that I had the pleasure of discharging him, my self from his bandages leather straps! and new set of teeth fills the void, made by a horse's foot, which almost dismembered his upper lip—Having been wedged under his dead horse shot under him, but before the fatal ball which did this mischief, it was first crimsoned by passing through the knee of its rider…

While he laid helpless from loss of blood, and wedged under his dead horse, another horse frantic from pain having been shot, plunged over him planting his fore foot over his upper lip from the base of the nose, completely carrying it away from the face, which hung to the cheek by a small fragment of flesh knocking out all his front teeth, out. When I journed to meet him, *he presented a pitiful sight—But after careful watching and constant attention, my noble and daring Son-in-law is now ready to resume Field duties—again—He is not discouraged by his experience in defense of his Flag—And is ready to front the enemy—as soon as he is permitted His younger brother whom I equipped for the Field was killed in battle, with two of my nephews! All three young Lieuts. Brave Boys! I glory to claim them my own dear flesh & blood—and I am proud to inform your Excellency that I still am honored by having yet three more nephews at this hour, on Field duty. And my errand is to put another in the field yet more nearer me still, my only Son, whose prayer to me is to get him also in the Army he is now twenty one years old and craves a commission to some Regiment. He is now on field duty, in capacity of clerkship. Left college to serve his country. I am a Stranger here, and if required to be formally presented I really know not to whom I can call upon....Please honor me with a line if it be possible I can call on your excellency, and when? Not with the crowd but alone, as I will be alone with my little Daughter.*

I have the honor to remain your Excellency's humble Servt

Mrs Col. Martin Burke
Washington, D.C.
February 1864

***

Our Most worthey presedent please Excuase Me for takeing this Liberty But I Cannot Express my Grate gratitude for your kindness in granting Me the order for My Son john H Bowden's of Chicago discharge what Goverment Bounty he has receved I have that Unbroken to refuned But the 1 hundred Dollers County Bounty I have Not Got It as I had to Use it Last winter to Maintain My Sick Boy and a dependant Sister I have Bin a widow Eleven years My Oldest Son a Loosing his health on Cheat Mountain Makes it Vary Bad for Us our kind president If you Can releave Me So that I Can take My Boy home with me I feel that God will reward you and I No he will Bless all your Undertakings please Answare Respectifully

Mrs Ann Bowden
Washington, D.C.
June 1864

***

On the first of this month my Son Eugene N.C. Promie, aged 17 years old, with two other lads were enticed by two men, offering them situations to Learn the Engineering in the United States navy, being taken to New York against my Will or consent, after arriving there they were forced into A Carriage, taken to Williamsburg to the Provost Marshall's Office, and there Sold as Substitutes in the Army (the men I learn having made Nineteen hundred dollars by the act) and immediately conveyed to Hart Island and from there sent to the front, his Father being in New York at the time my Son desired to see him, to get his consent, as that was the provision made, but was not allowed, but was forced away as before stated by threats, the Men are now in Prison for Abduction. My poor boy I have just received A Letter from who is now in the Chesapeake Hospital Sick and expected to be sent away; My Dear Boy is just from College inexperienced and but a Child

And Oh! let not the appeal of a Mothers Grief be in Vain I am unable through my distressed feelings to dictate to you A more appealing letter…not the appeal of A Sorrowful Mother be in Vain…Hoping the Prayer of A Mother may be heard through you and my Son restored to me

I remain your Esteemed Friend

Amanda A Promie
Philadelphia
June 1864

***

Mr Lincoln

Allow me to congratulate you on your re-election. It is certainly a very great compliment to be invited to preside over the destinies of a great nation—a second term.…You have never refused me any thing I have asked—I hope I have not been unreasonable—or imposed on your naturally kind benevolent disposition. I have a young son—Lemuel S. Hardin—who has been a short time in the Southern Army—has been severely wounded—he has made his way through the lines—and is now in Canada—He is crippled for life—and is anxious to return to his home and family—He has been a resident for the last three years in Louisville Ky…

After a young man has—"sown his wild oats"—or—"seen the elephant"—he is often better prepared to settle down and become a sensible man—he has a better appreciation of home and the advantage of a good position. Mr President—I claim your indulgence in favor of my petition—not on the merit of the case—but as an act of clemency to a wayward youth—My waif of a son is endowed with many of the good qualities of the noble man from which he comes—both of head and heart.

Yours respectfully—S.E. Walworth
December 1864

***

To his Excellency Abraham Lincoln:

Sir,

A sick and almost heartbroken mother again sentenced to make another appeal to you for the release of her dear son, Samuel Hardinge Jr., who, through gross misrepresentation and exaggeration on the part of enemies, was first confined in Carroll Prison; and afterward, without being allowed to vindicate his own innocence, transferred to Fort Delaware. [Hardinge was the husband of Belle Boyd, a Confederate spy.] *In the only letters which I have received from him since he has been there, he thus writes: "Oh My God! How long am I to remain in this horrible place, full of rebels and secessionists. Oh my parents! Do all you possibly can to get me out of here. My God! My poor wife in England! She tells me in a letter—'For God's sake to send her some money!' And I in prison! Why should they put me in here! I who have taken the oath of allegiance to the U.S. Government and who have never done anything against it. Oh it is hard! And I pray God daily and nightly that President Lincoln may grant my release!"*

I transcribe his own words that you may see what his real feelings are. I told you, sir, in my recent interview with you, that he might, so far as I know, have been guilty of some small utterances, smarting as he was under the unfair and cruel suspicions cast upon him in the affair of the "Greyhound"; but, guilty of a single act against the good of his country—never! You, sir, can judge for yourself whether or not this is the language of a foe to the Government. Oh President Lincoln! I implore and entreat of you to grant my son's release! My health is rapidly failing under this dreadful blow! I appeal to your kindly nature!…When you think of the magnificent glorious Christmas gift which General Sherman presented to you, will you not confer upon a poor heartbroken mother, the—to you, small—News Years gift of the liberty of her dear son.

Sarah A.M. Hardinge
Brooklyn, New York
January 1865

***

Honble Abraham Lincoln
President of the U.S. America

I have heard from good authority that if I suppress the Book I have now ready for publication, you may be induced to consider leniently the case of my husband, S. Wylde Hardinge, now a prisoner in Fort Delaware, I think it would be well for you & me to come to some definite understanding. My Book was originally not intended to be more than a personal narrative, but since my husband's unjust arrest I had intended making it political, & had introduced many atrocious circumstances respecting your government with which I am so well acquainted & which would open the eyes of Europe to many things of which the world on this side of the water little dreams. If you will release my husband & set him free, so that he may join me here in England by the beginning of March—I pledge you my word that my Book shall be suppressed. Should my husband not be with me by the 25th of March I shall at once place my Book in the hands of a publisher.

Trusting an immediate reply,
I am Sir, Yr. Obdt. Sevt.
Belle Boyd Hardinge
England
January 1865[208]

6

EPILOGUE AND CONCLUSION

The history of trauma during the Civil War is an area of exploration that is truly a work in progress. This book hopes to be a helpful addition to the discourse, inspiring further research and discussion. There is a growing body of research regarding intergenerational transmission of trauma and pain. Has the pain experienced by those who served in various capacities during the war been imprinted on the psyche of our society in modern times? Are some of the issues we currently deal with, including drug addiction, ongoing trauma and pain, a vestige of the 1860s? How do we as a nation deal with trauma of those from over 150 years ago, trauma that may still have an impact today?

Since the Civil War, we have learned the importance of supporting families of those killed in a meaningful way. According to the organization Operation 300:

> *We believe that when a member of our armed services gives his life in defense of our great nation, the least we can do is pledge to honor that sacrifice by caring for his family. This is the heart behind Operation 300, a registered 501c3 not for profit organization which hosts adventure camps for children who have lost their fathers as a result of military service, pairing each child with a father-aged male mentor who spends the weekend doing things with the children they might have done with their Dad.*[209]

What can we conclude about trauma, healing and the Civil War? First, PTSD exists, and there are modern-day, long-term consequences; some of these consequences may have origins in the Civil War. With respect to long-term, modern-day consequences of PTSD, the article "Cognitive Deficits Are Common in Veterans with Parkinson's Disease" posits:[210]

> *Among veterans with Parkinson's disease 46.9% have a cognitive-related diagnosis, and African Americans have a higher rate of such diagnoses than Caucasians, according to research reported at the 66th Annual meeting of the American Academy of Neurology. Race, Agent Orange Exposure, a history of traumatic brain injury (TBI) and a history of post-traumatic stress disorder (PTSD) were the factors associated with a higher rate of cognitive diagnosis.*[211]

Brandon Barton, MD, a neurologist at the Jesse Brown VA Medical Center in Chicago, analyzed data for veterans with Parkinson's disease. "VA databases are large, well organized, and provide access to subject identification and health history in a unique way that is not otherwise available in other health care systems" notes Dr. Barton. "We hypothesized that veterans with Parkinson's disease have a high prevalence of cognitive deficits and those with any of the three target exposures [Agent Orange, TBI and PTSD] have more frequent cognitive diagnoses than those without exposure."

With respect to the Civil War specifically, according to author Pizarro, "Unfortunately, it is likely that the deleterious health effects seen in [the Civil War] are applicable to health and well-being of soldiers fighting wars in the 21st century."[212]

Second, our country currently has a dire drug addiction epidemic. While researchers and historians can debate the origins of this current crisis, the Civil War can certainly offer insights that may be helpful from a comparison standpoint.

Pain is the main reason most people present to the emergency room; however, "[i]t is what happens after patients leave the emergency department (ED) that public health experts believe has contributed to a crisis of addiction in the United States." When patients are discharged, their pain management frequently involves a prescription for opioids. These pain medications are then refilled by a family practitioner. Since the medication has kept pain at bay, they seek refills from their primary doctors. While a small number of opioid prescriptions are filled by way of the ER, the Emergency Department is often viewed as the gateway to pain medication addiction.

Third, while soldiers suffered greatly during the war, others experienced trauma in ways that were long-lasting and detrimental. In healthcare workers to families and friends, the psychological damage left in the wake of the war was far-reaching.

Fourth, the advocacy efforts around the war specifically for getting help for those suffering after the war were formidable and long lasting. Clara Barton's work with the Red Cross is one of the more visible examples, but everyday people writing letters to officials, public health workers and politicians all contributed to shining a light on these issues.

Fifth, New York and Washington, D.C., were invaluable in leading the efforts for hospital care and homes for veterans during and after the Civil War. From Bellevue to Howard University to New York Presbyterian and the Bath Veterans Affairs Hospital, institutions continue to provide critical care to those in need.

Finally, recovery from trauma is something that requires all of society to band together to help those in need. In her book *Trauma and Recovery*, Herman speaks about the courage that a society as a whole must embrace in order to face the atrocities perpetrated by some of its members. It is this courage that Americans as a whole will need in order to deal with the continuing physical, emotional and interpersonal impact of PTSD, which affects all Americans.[213] The Civil War demonstrates examples of support for others. We as a nation need to continue these efforts, being vigilant in supporting trauma care and trauma recovery.

The title of this book is *Healing Civil War Veterans in New York and Washington, D.C.* Healing can come in many forms. We can heal ourselves through caring for others as in the case of Dr. Alexander Augusta. Clara Barton healed thousands of widows and families searching for veterans after the war. Lewis H. Douglass healed a community of veterans through his advocacy and writing. In the end, while the pain of the war stayed with many veterans, their ability to heal themselves and others is their lasting, beautiful, enduring legacy.

NOTES

Introduction

1. de Jong, et al., "Lifetime Events and Posttraumatic Stress Disorder," 555–62. According to de Jong et al., PTSD is the most commonly reported psychiatric disorder resulting from experiencing a traumatic event; "Discrimination is defined in civil rights law as unfavorable or unfair treatment of a person or class of persons in comparison to others who are not members of the protected class because of race, sex, color, religion, national origin, age, physical/mental handicap, sexual harassment, sexual orientation or reprisal for opposition to discriminatory practices or participation in the EEO process"; according to the OHRP (Office of Health Research and Policy), "[I]n epidemiological studies, the investigator is attempting to identify risk factors for particular diseases, conditions, or behaviors. Or risks that result from particular causes, such as environmental or industrial agents."; Hidalgo and Davidson, "Post Traumatic Stress Disorder," 5; de Girolamo and Mcfarlane, "Epidemiology of PTSD," 33.
2. de Jong, "Lifetime Events and Posttraumatic Stress Disorder," 555–62.
3. Ibid.
4. The abbreviation "PTSD" will be used throughout the book to be consistent with the 2013 DSM-5.

Chapter 1

5. Trimble, *Post-traumatic Neurosis*, 940–41.
6. Chadwick, "Mental Trauma," www.npr.org/templates/story/story.php?storyId=5194224.
7. Ford, "Suffering in Silence."
8. Ibid.
9. Ibid.
10. Ibid.
11. Ibid.

12. Friedman, "History of PTSD."

13. U.S. Department of Veterans Affairs, "PTSD Basics," PTSD: National Center for PTSD, www.ptsd.va.gov/understand/what/ptsd_basics.asp.

14. Ibid.

15. Yehuda, "Post-Traumatic Stress Disorder," 108. Yehuda states that "[t]o be given a diagnosis of PTSD, a person has to have been exposed to an extreme stressor or traumatic event to which he or she responded with fear, helplessness, or horror and to have three distinct types of symptoms consisting of re-experiencing of the event, avoidance of reminders of the event, and hyper arousal for at least one month."

16. Nordenberg, "Escaping the Prison."

17. Lamberg, "Psychiatrists Explore Legacy," 523. See also Clark, "Posttraumatic Stress Disorder," 28: "PTSD can range from acute PTSD, with symptoms manifesting after 3 months, to chronic PTSD manifesting for 3 months or longer to delayed onset where symptoms appear at least 6 months after the traumatic event."

18. Lamberg, "Psychiatrists Explore Legacy," 523.

19. Ibid.

20. de Girolamo and Mcfarlane, "Epidemiology of PTSD," 36.

21. Ibid., 35.

22. Gorrell, "Noah Wyle and Real Life Trauma," 32. See also Breslau, et al., "Short Screening Scale," 6.

23. Breslau, et al., "Previous Exposure to Trauma."

24. Hidalgo and Davidson, "Post Traumatic Stress Disorder," 6. An added wrinkle to the stressor issue is the passage of time and the age of the individual being evaluated. According to Dr. Peter Ziarnowski, "Any stressor in life—a death in the family—a new job may stir emotions....Retirement may present a problem. PTSD may have been like a wave that—like a surfer—you could ride and stay ahead of when you were younger. But as you get older, the wave catches up to you."

25. Ibid.

26. Ibid.

27. Ibid. "There were circumstances beyond exposure to combat in which a soldier could become a sufferer of PTSD. The unimaginable horrors endured by those who were captured—or gobbled as the saying went and sent to prisoner of war camps often exceeded those of combat. Many captured soldiers on both sides considered remand to a prison camp tantamount to a death sentence; even if they survived, they were often physically and psychologically damaged for life. Sometimes the most basic functions relating to a solder's life could induce PTSD symptoms. Infantry soldiers in the Civil War generally traveled by foot, conceivably covering thousands of miles during the course of their service. Marching, while a deceptively simple task on the surface, frequently presented hardships for which the soldiers were ill-prepared. Military physicians were mandated as part of their responsibilities, to recognize and diagnose mental disorders among the troops. The science of psychology was still years in the future, however, and generally neither the military hierarchy nor the medical profession understood, or was disposed to make allowances for soldiers whose experience in war had mentally incapacitated them. The symptoms were frequently not recorded or were improperly identified or commonly dismissed with such facile diagnoses as acute mania 'soldiers heart' nervous shock railway brain melancholy nostalgia dementia hysteria feeble will moral turpitude cowardice. The responsibility for caring for those affected by PTSD generally fell upon the victim's families depending on the symptoms exhibited by the suffering veteran this could be a frustrating and at times impossible task. Those affected often took to drink, which frequently led to

violence. Insomnia was not uncommon, with the sufferer dazedly roaming the house or yard. This could turn frightening should he be armed and looking for an imaginary foe. Medical records and family accounts provide numerous accounts of troubled veterans who slept with a gun, knife, or ax for protection against 'enemy attack.' Ultimately unable to cope and with no end in sight, the family would have little choice but to have him 'committed' to an already overcrowded state or county mental facility."

28. Ibid. "Firearm technology during the Civil War saw the widespread use of the Minié ball, a French development that wasn't a ball at all but a hollow-based conical soft-lead projectile typically ranging from .58 to .69 caliber. Whereas a standard musket ball might break a bone in its course, the Minié ball tended to shatter bone and pulverize flesh, to the extent that an affected limb normally had to be amputated. Even in cases where the arm or leg might be saved, the surgeons were so overworked—and in some cases, unskilled— that amputation became the standard treatment. Shock from the procedure itself killed a number of soldiers. Those who survived faced the likelihood of infection, since the concept of sterilizing instruments or even the routine washing of hands was still years in the future. Some soldiers who lived through the operation found themselves addicted to the morphine or opium to ease the pain. For those who survived the surgery, the homecoming itself offered its own kind of nightmare, exacerbating the stressors under which a victim of PTSD was already suffering. Most soldiers had made their living through physical labor prior to the war. Whether a man had been a farmer or factory hand or teamster or construction worker, blacksmith or coal miner, the loss of a limb signified the end of his livelihood. His options were few: a state-run solders' home, the county poorhouse or the street. For an already traumatized veteran finding himself crippled, unemployed and unable to support himself or his family reduced to beginning or living on the dole, the psychological impact was devastating."

29. American Psychiatric Association, "Posttraumatic Stress Disorder."

30. *American Heritage Dictionary*.

31. Hirsch, *Cultural Literacy*, 325.

32. Scurfield, "Positive and Negative Aspects." Scurfield goes on to state that "[t]he nature of exposure to race-related experiences may have been: (a) discrete and markedly memorable events, single-incident or repetitive; (b) more covert or subtle exposure; or (c) cumulative/ repetitive over a period of time. The concept of insidious exposure is very important—a more chronic, pervasive type of exposure to years of racist-oriented attitudes and behaviors; however, no one episode may be sufficient to meet the DSM-IV TR adjustment and stress disorder diagnostic criteria."

33. Faison, in *Racism* (177), asserts, "Racism will be present in America as long as there are black people in America and white people in America. It would seem that blacks would be keenly aware of this by now and would be doing something constructive about it. If dying for the right to vote, educating themselves, getting lighter skin and longer hair, and acting white hasn't changed things in the last hundred years, it seems blacks would be ready to try something else"; "Only the insensitive white American can be surprised to hear that 'all blacks are angry.' To believe otherwise given the blacks' history in America surely is to reveal a psychological obtuseness of the greatest proportions"; Baughman, *Black Americans*, 57.

34. Hirsch, *Cultural Literacy*, 315.

35. Ibid., 318.

36. Ibid., 209.

37. Ibid.

38. Ibid.

39. National Violence Against Women Prevention Center, https://mainweb-v.musc.edu/vawprevention.
40. Herman, *Trauma and Recovery*, 243–44.
41. Rich, "Primary Care."
42. Butts, "Black Mask of Humanity," 339.
43. Hirsch, *Cultural Literacy*, 210. There is a link between being African American and developing PTSD. The African American's experience of traumatic stress is often characterized by greater exposure to stressors and more long-term averse effects. This is only exacerbated by the lack of economic resources, racism and prejudice.
44. Friedman, "History of PTSD in Veterans," www.ptsd.va.gov/understand/what/history_ptsd.asp.
45. U.S. Department of Veterans Affairs, "PTSD Basics."
46. Meisler, "Trauma, PTSD and Substance Abuse."
47. van der Kolk, "Assessment and Treatment." Van der Kolk elucidates on the issue of PTSD and interpersonal difficulties, stating, "Over the years, it has become clear that in clinical settings the majority of traumatized treatment seeking patients suffer from a variety of psychological problems that are not included in the diagnosis of PTSD. These include depression and self-hatred. dissociation and depersonalization, aggressive behavior against self and others, problems with intimacy and impairment in the capacity to experience pleasure, satisfaction and 'fun.' Many of these problems that are not categorized under the rubric of PTSD are often classified as 'co-morbid conditions,' rather than being recognized as part of a spectrum of trauma."
48. de Girolamo and Mcfarlane, "Epidemiology of PTSD," 46.
49. U.S. Department of Veterans Affairs, "PTSD Basics." Racial discrimination compared to life stress and demographic variables was also studied in African Americans, as it predicted psychiatric disorders.
50. U.S. Department of Veterans Affairs, "PTSD General Facts."
51. Ibid.
52. In the New York case of Portee v. Hastava, 863 F. Supp. 597 (EDNY 1994), Paul, Donna and Justin Portee sued Hastava Real Estate, and Henry M. Hastava M. Hastava and Benjamin Vajda individually, for Title VIII violations of civil rights. The Portees, an interracial couple with one child, Justin, decided to find a new home in 1989. Mrs. Portee saw an advertisement in New York's *Newsday* magazine placed by Hastava Real Estate for a house in New York. Mrs. Portee went back to the real estate office with Mr. Vajda and obtained the key for the signed lease and wrote out checks for the apartment. Mr. Vajda requested that Mr. Portee come by the office to sign the lease. Mrs. Portee proceeded to take Mr. Portee first by the premises and that same day to the office. According to Mr. Portee, when he and his wife entered the HRE offices, Mr. Vajda became "very nervous" and "went upstairs for about 10 or 15 minutes." According to Mr. Portee, when Mr. Vajda returned from upstairs, he told the Portees that he didn't have the lease, then grabbed the key from Mr. Portee. At this point, according to the Portees, there was more "back and forth" until the Portees finally asked for their checks back. Mr. Vajda stated that he did not have their checks. Justin, who had been present during the entire exchange, asked his parents what was happening. His father testified that he told his son Mr. Vajda was a bigot who would not rent to them and "[because I'm black]." Mr. Vajda's account obviously differs from this account. Mrs. Portee told their son HRE would not rent to them "because of your father." The Portees immediately contacted legal counsel to ascertain their rights. According to the testimony from Mrs. Portee, after the incident, she was "upset," and her work suffered. "She could not concentrate on simple tasks, and she was very nervous.

She made many little mistakes at work." Coworkers confirmed that, for a period of one to two months, following the incident at HRE, Mrs. Portee was "not herself." As for Justin, according to the testimony, he was very excited about the potential move. After the incident at the real estate agency, according to his mother, he "cried a little." It is interesting to note that the Portee family had been involved in a fire in their building during this time, thus they were experiencing a number of different traumatic events during this time. Mr. Portee's symptoms were the most prominent of the three plaintiffs. He testified that immediately after the incident he felt "low, like I was a low-life animal." Since the HRE event, Mr. Portee testified to "[a] dep [*sic*] hurt , very dep [*sic*] hurt. Lord it hur [*sic*] where it comes to my son and I'm trying to give my son what he want and somebody tries to take it away from me…when I try to do for my son and people tell me I can't have it because I'm black.…It's very hard." Mr. Portee also described increased alcohol intake and decreased social activity. "I used to go to parties with [Mrs. Portee], have a good time, one or two drinks, dance. Now we don't even do that no more.…I don't feel like being with people no more. It turned me against them…I still feel bad, low." After a jury trial, the jury returned a verdict for the plaintiff awarding general compensatory damages, and interestingly, emotional damages were awarded by the jury in the amount of $100,000 for Mrs. Portee, $100,000 for Mr. Portee and $80,000 for Justin Portee.

53. Kessler, "Posttraumatic Stress Disorder," 61.
54. Breslau et al., "Traumatic Events and Posttraumatic Stress," 216–22.
55. Kessler, "Posttraumatic Stress Disorder," 61. The report goes on to state that "racism, discrimination and prejudice place Blacks at great risk for reduced mental health status. Blacks at all levels of socioeconomic status are more likely to have access to fewer economic. social and political resources and to be affected by institutional racism which…place them at increased risk for the development of some mental disorders."
56. Kessler et al., "Epidemiological Risk Factors," 23–59.
57. Prigerson, "Population Attributable Fractions," 59–63.
58. Bromet, "Risk Factors," 355. The five other, more uncommon events were: direct combat experience in war; involvement in a fire, flood or natural disaster; threatened with a weapon, held captive or kidnapped; suffered a great shock because one of the events on this list happened to someone close to you; or experienced some other terrible experience "that most people never go through."
59. Osofsky, "Effects of Exposure."
60. Lamberg, "Psychiatrists Explore Legacy," 523. Interestingly, it is only as children mature that they begin to understand the impact of their childhood traumas. Because of this trauma, adults who experienced trauma as children are more susceptible to further traumatic events.
61. Breslau et al., "Traumatic Events and Posttraumatic Stress," 216–22.
62. Compas et al., "Coping With Stress."
63. Breslau et al., "Short Screening Scale," 156:6. According to Breslau, "[C]hildhood trauma increased the risk that a new trauma experienced in adulthood would lead to PTSD."
64. Ibid.
65. Bromet, "Risk Factors," 360.
66. Gorrell, "Noah Wyle," 32.
67. U.S. Department of Health and Human Services. "Facing Addiction in America."
68. Kessler, "Posttraumatic Stress Disorder," 89.
69. Butts, "The Black Mask of Humanity," 339
70. Kessler, "Posttraumatic Stress Disorder," 89.
71. Ibid.

72. Novae, "Traumatic Stress."
73. Research on Holocaust offspring can be a productive model for establishing research parameters in other areas.
74. Hirsch, *Cultural Literacy*, 118.
75. Ibid., 123.
76. de Girolamo and Mcfarlane, "Epidemiology of PTSD," 896–902.
77. U.S. Department of Health and Human Services, "Facing Addiction in America."
78. Hirsch, *Cultural Literacy*, 227.
79. Kessler, "Posttraumatic Stress Disorder," 61.
80. Ibid.
81. Yehuda, "Post-Traumatic Stress Disorder," 108.
82. Kessler, "Posttraumatic Stress Disorder," 61.

Chapter 2

83. Winston, "Smith, Sylvanus," http://www.blackpast.org/aah/sylvanus-smith-1831-1911.
84. Ibid.
85. Ibid.
86. Ibid.
87. Ibid.
88. "Susan M. Steward," www.encyclopedia.com/history/encyclopedias-almanacs-transcripts-and-maps/steward-susan-mckinney; MacLean, "Susan McKinney Steward," http://civilwarrx.blogspot.com/2016/05/susan-mckinney-steward-first-african.html.
89. Malinenko, "Susan Smith McKinney Steward," www.bklynlibrary.org/blog/2018/01/25/Susan-smith-mckinney.
90. Cook, "Dying to Get Home," http://warfarehistorynetwork.com/daily/civil-war/dying-to-get-home-ptsd-in-the-civil-war.
91. Ibid.
92. "Second Annual Report of the Women's Central Association of Relief." For example, the WCAR and Sanitary Commission established a directory early in the war with the names of all patients in New York, New Jersey, New England, Washington, Philadelphia and Louisville. This list also included their statuses and conditions. It was critical for relieving relatives of anxiety regarding loved ones and also helped relatives locate injured soldiers. U.S. Department of Health and Human Services, collections.nlm.nih.gov/catalog/Mom:nlmuid-101181516-bk.
93. Brace and Donaldson, *Life of Charles Loring Brace*, 248.
94 "Second Annual Report."
95. Ibid.
96. Cook, "Dying to Get Home," http://warfarehistorynetwork.com/daily/civil-war/dying-to-get-home-ptsd-in-the-civil-war.
97. Ibid.
98. Ibid.
99. Ibid.
100. Ibid.
101. Jones, "Invisible Wounds."
102. Ibid. "By the morning of April 25, 1861, residents of Washington had been expecting a Confederate attack for almost two weeks; for the last five days, the city had been completely cut off from the rest of the nation. No trains. No traffic into the city. No telegraph. No

mail. Only the morning before at the White House, a despondent President Lincoln had greeted the wounded soldiers of the Sixth Massachusetts—the last reinforcements to arrive since April 19—telling them, 'I don't believe there is any North. The Seventh Regiment is a myth.' Suddenly, the long-delayed Seventh New York volunteers finally arrived at the B&O station, and the nation's capital was saved. 'And now a thousand voices,' exulted the *New York World*, 'shouted with one acclaim: "It's the Seventh Regiment!"' David Carll served as a private with Company I Twenty-Sixth United States Colored Infantry in the Civil War. He enlisted on January 2, 1864, at Jamaica, New York. The regiment was organized at Riker's Island (located in the East River) on February 27, 1864. He was later deployed to Beaufort, South Carolina. He was discharged on August 28, 1865, at Oyster Bay. With his enlistment bounty of $300 he was able to buy a $200 parcel of land in Oyster Bay, New York, on January 7, 1864. David Carll was married to Louisa. He was the father of Herbert, Frank, Wilbur, Cassie, Armenia, Herman, Agnes and Josie. He later remarried; his second wife was named Julia. He dropped the second *L* from his last name, and subsequent generations continued to use that spelling."

103. Ibid.

104. Ibid.

105. American Battlefield Trust, "Georgeanna Woolsey," www.civilwar.org/learn/articles/georgeanna-woolsey-day-life-northern-nurse.

Chapter 3

106. Ford, "Suffering in Silence."

107. Soodalter, "Shock of War," www.historynet.com/the-shock-of-War.htm.

108. Jones, "Invisible Wounds."

109. Ibid.

110. Ibid.

111. Pizarro, "Physical and Mental Health Costs," 193–200.

112. Ibid.

113. Ibid.

114. Ibid.

115. Ibid. Limitation on study: "Because not all signs and symptoms of cardiovascular heart disease or PTSD were assessed, veterans are not assumed to have had these diagnoses. Nonetheless, although we are unable [to] construct current medical diagnoses as outcome variables using this dataset, Civil War era physicians were able to recognize and record signs of physical and mental disease that are indicative of modern diagnoses."

116. Ibid.

117. Ford, "Suffering in Silence." Note: While not a D.C. or New York story, author Sarah Ford tells the story of Dr. William Chester Minor in such a compelling fashion that it deserves mention: "Dr. William Chester Minor was a surgeon in the Union Army for several years. Minor served at various battles including the Battle of the Wilderness, one of the most gruesome conflicts of the entire war. As a surgeon, Dr. Minor had seen the worst that war had to offer. He had experienced delusions and paranoid fits after the war and as a result, Minor was diagnosed with soldier's heart, an early form of PTSD. In August of eighteen seventy-two, Minor shot and killed a man in the streets of London, England. According to his testimony, Minor claimed he had been experiencing a delusion where he was back on the battlefield and the man was an enemy soldier trying to kill him. The courts found him not guilty by reason of insanity and he was sent to Broadmoor Hospital, a notorious insane asylum in Crownthrone, England. Arguably one of the most intrusive

symptoms of PTSD are flashbacks. The person is experiencing an illusion or vision of the past trauma. They are essentially re-living the event allowing them to experience it all over again. Minor may have truly believed he was back on that battlefield and was fighting to preserve his life. William Minor's incident could have been a result of post-traumatic stress disorder from his combat experience."

118. Ibid.

119. Yale School of Public Health, "Dr. Cortlandt Van Rensselaer Creed." "Cortlandt Van Resselaer Creed, MD 1857, the first African American graduate of Yale Medical School, was the first person of African descent to receive a degree in any discipline from Yale. Only a very small number of African Americans had previously received medical degrees from U.S. institutions before Dr. Creed, and none from the Ivy schools. His Yale MD thesis was entitled 'On the Blood'—a discourse on the physiology and chemistry of blood and circulation. Despite what Dr. Creed described in one of his letters to Douglas as a prevailing national sentiment of 'prejudice against color,' he reported, 'I never experienced any other than the most polite treatment from my fellow class-mates.' Dr. Creed remained in New Haven after graduation from Yale and developed a large, successful, ethnically-mixed medical practice. At the outbreak of the Civil War, he wrote to Connecticut Governor Buckingham requesting a commission to serve, but was refused because of his race. In 1863, President Lincoln authorized the recruitment of African American troops and the Connecticut governor issued a call to arms to men of color. Creed wrote, 'On every side we behold colored sons rallying to the sound of Liberty and Union.' He was appointed 1st Lieutenant and Surgeon of the 31st Regiment U.S. Colored Troops 1864 (30th Connecticut Volunteer Infantry Regiment) and served until the end of the Civil War.

Dr. Creed married Drucilla Wright with whom he had four sons. After her death, he married Mary Paul of Brooklyn, New York with whom he had six children. He briefly practiced in New York but returned to New Haven for the rest of his career. Cited frequently in the local news and the *New York Times* for his medical and forensic skills, he was consulted for a surgical opinion at the time of President Garfield's assassination.

Dr. Creed died from 'Bright's disease' on August 8th, 1900 and was buried in the family plot in Grove Street Cemetery." Wikipedia, "31st Infantry Regiment." The Thirty-First Infantry was an African American regiment raised at Hart's Island on April 29, 1864. It was active as of November 14, 1864. In May 1864, it merged with the Thirtieth Connecticut Colored Volunteers. The commanding officer was Colonel Henry C. Ward, and the unit was mustered out in November 1865.

120. Cordingley and Denbow, "Pioneer African-American Physicians." Dr. Elliott was born a slave in Greenup County, Kentucky, on March 10, 1826. During the Civil War (1861–65), he served as a hospital steward in the Twenty-Sixth United States Colored Infantry. This rank seems to have combined some of the functions of modern hospital administrators, pharmacists, dentists, physicians and nurses.

121. Elliott, "African American Pioneer Physician."

122. Evans, "Remembering."

123. Karppi, "African American Civil War Museum Honors OB Civil Vet David Carll."

124. Ibid.

125. America Civil War Soldier Letters Home, www.americancivilwar.com/kids_zone/soldiers_letters_civil_war.html.

126. Ibid.

127. Ibid.

128. Ibid.

129. Gilder Lehrman, "Donahue, Thomas (fl. 1863) to Almira Winchell," www.gilderlehrman. org/content/almira-winchell-3.

130. Lively, "JE Hanger Lost."

131. For additional information about Chinese American heroes, please visit the Chinese American Heroes website at www.scmp.com/magazines/post-magazine/ article/1270170/gettysburg-redress.

132. Library of Congress, "Sergeant Cornelius V. Moore of Company B, 100th New York Volunteers, a Sergeant of 39th Illinois Regiment, a Corporal of 106th New York Volunteers, and a Private of the 11th Vermont Regiment, http://hdl.loc.gov/loc.pnp/ ppmsca.30571"; Envelope from Cornelius Moore, LOT 14043, http://hdl.loc.gov/loc. pnp/ppmsca.33801.

133. Ibid.

134. Ibid.

135. Ibid.

136. Ibid. Discharge form for Cornelius Moore, 1865, http://hdl.loc.gov/loc.pnp/ ppmsca.33802.

137. SUNY Morrisville, "Civil War Letters."

138. Ibid.

139. Ibid.

140. Civil War Home Page, "Sullivan Ballou's Letter."

141 Butts, *African American Medicine*, 53.

142 Wooster, "Diary of Lewis Bramer, Jr."

143. U.S. Senate, "Clara Barton and Senator Henry Wilson."

144. Ford, "Suffering in Silence."

145. Ibid.

146. Ibid.

147. Ibid. "Arguably one of the most intense contributing factors to psychological effects and disorders were the prisoner of war (P.O.W.) camps. Some of the most detestable incidences in the war occurred inside these camps. Psychologically, people are put in situations with numerous traumas, such as ubiquitous death, fighting and abuse, making P.O.W camps a minefield for psychological disorders. Camps like Salisbury, Libby, Douglas and the most notorious Andersonville were overpopulated and did not have proper supplies for the number of prisoners it contained. At one point, Andersonville detained thirty-two thousand men but the original capacity was for only ten thousand men. When Sherman's soldiers liberated Andersonville, they found some prisoners completely emaciated. At the end of the war when supplies were scarce, rations were withheld. 'No rations issued yesterday to any of the prisoners and a third of all here are on the very point of starvation…' Prisoners would fight, even kill, other prisoners for whatever they might have in their possession that could aid in their survival. 'Have just seen a big fight among the prisoners; just like so many snarly dogs, cross and peevish.' The fight to survive in hellish places like Andersonville, Libby, Salisbury and Douglas was exceedingly stressful. Witnessing the intense trauma of death on a daily basis was more than enough to produce PTSD."

148. Ibid.

149. Ibid.

150. Cook, "Dying to Get Home."

151. Ibid.

152. Ibid.

153. Ibid.

154. Ford, "Suffering in Silence."

155. Ibid.
156. Greenhagen, "Emerson Clark."
157. Ibid.
158. Horowitz, "Did Civil War Soldiers Have PTSD?."
159. Ibid.
160 Ibid.
161. Carter, *Mind of a Negro*, 544.
162. Douglass, *Narrative of the Life*, 245.
163. Wills, *Die Free*, 69.

Chapter 4

164. Clara Barton Missing Soldier Museum, www.clarabartonmuseum.org.
165. Ibid.
166. Ibid.
167. Ibid.
168. Ibid.
169. www.westadsa.org/cms/li68/id01904074/centricIty/Domain/2734/shaw%20letter. docx.
170. Moore, *Rebellion Record*, 25–62.
171. Ibid.
172. MacLean, "Annie Haggerty Shaw."
173. Street, "Under the Influence."
174. Ibid.
175. Ibid.
176. Ibid.
177. Ibid.
178. Ibid.
179. Ibid.
180. Ibid.
181. Ford, "Suffering in Silence."
182. Ibid.
183. Ibid.
184. Ibid.
185. Ibid.
186. O'Brien, *My Life*.
187. Ford, "Suffering in Silence."
188. Shepard, *Now or Never*, 31.
189. The Home for Little Wanderers, www.thehome.org.
190. Brace and Donaldson, *Life of Charles Loring Brace*, 256.
191. Fynes, "Orphanage for Children."

Chapter 5

192. Cook, "Dying to Get Home." "In May 1864, Civil War was still raging in our land, although the Confederacy was approaching its collapse, emancipation had taken place and the ex-salves were crowding into the Union Army. It was at this eventful time that the General Conference of the African Methodist Episcopal Church met in Philadelphia,

assembling in old Bethel Church. From Hilton Head I proceeded to Beaufort, about 16 miles distance from the 'head' (as we soon learned to call the headquarter post); situated on Beaufort River, landing there May 27, 1865. Here, inexperienced, unaccustomed to the climate, and entirely unprepared to cope with the topsy-turvy conditions I met, I began my work. I began at the beginning; by securing board temporarily with a Mrs. Beam who kept a kind of officers' mess where were boarding Major Augusta Chief surgeon of one of the colored regiments, and who was in fact the first colored man to out one officers' uniform in the Union Army during the Civil War and from whose shoulders ruffians tore the straps in Baltimore; Captain O.S.B. Wall, and a number of Civilians. I did not remain in this public house but soon after found board with a lady named Cruz from Palatka, Fla. She and her daughter kept a very pleasant home and here I and Major Martin R. Delaney boarded. I visited the sick and buried the dead, and finally got together and organized a church. A brother had been preaching there before, under the supervision of our church had not been organized. Hence I did not begin my formal work as pastor of a mission church until June 18, 1865."

193. Deeben, "Caring for Veterans."

194. Ibid.

195. Ibid.

196. Ibid.

197. Starr, "Social Transformation of American Medicine," 169.

198 Palmer, "Floating Hospital."

199. Bath VA Medical Center, "125th Anniversary Booklet," https://www.bath.va.gov/docs/125thbooklet.pdf.

200. Ibid. Washington was often inundated with casualties from the Army of the Potomac. Historian Flood wrote:

"Steamboats with names like Lizzie Baker, Connecticut, and General Hooker, their whistles blaring in harsh ghostly tones, landed at the Sixth Street wharves in downtown Washington, where long lines of horse drawn ambulances waited to take the wounded to Washington's twenty-one overcrowded hospitals." Mary Clemmer Ames, a Washington resident during the Civil War, wrote: "Arid hill, and sodden plain showed alike the horrid trail of war. Forts bristled above every hill-top. Soldiers were entrenched at every gate-way. Shed hospitals covered acres on acres in every suburb. Churches, art-halls and private mansions were filled with the wounded and dying of the American armies. The endless roll of the army wagon seemed never still. The rattle of the anguish-laden ambulance, the piercing cries of the sufferers…made morning, noon and night too dreadful to be borne."

201. Ibid.

202. Ibid.

203. Ibid.

204. Ibid.

205. Ibid.

206. Ibid.

207. On March 17, 1865, John Wilkes Booth learned that President Lincoln planned to visit wounded soldiers at Campbell General Hospital and attend a performance of the play *Still Waters Run Deep* in the theater there. Historian Robert H. Fowler wrote: "With an hour's notice, according to John Surratt, the gang raced out, waited until they saw a carriage approach. Riding alongside, they saw the man in the vehicle was not Lincoln. It may have been Salmon P. Chase, the Chief Justice of the Supreme Court, who did attend the show." President Lincoln had changed his schedule, thus postponing his assassination for nearly a month.

208. Burlingame, *Inner World*; Holzer, *Dear Mr. Lincoln*; Sigaud, "When Belle Boyd Wrote Lincoln"; Library of Congress, Abraham Lincoln Papers. Lincoln made no notation on Belle's letter, nor did he indicate any knowledge of the "atrocious circumstances" to which she referred. Perhaps because the war was almost over, perhaps because Samuel Hardinge's only crime was being Belle's husband, perhaps because the president admired the Rebel girl's audacity, the prisoner was released on February 3, ten days after Belle made her demand. She would name her baby daughter Grace and, later, her son Arthur Davis Lee Jackson, after her favorite Confederate heroes.

Chapter 6

209. Operation 300, www.operation300.com.
210. Barton, "Cognitive Deficits," 32.
211. Ibid.
212. Pizarro, "Physical and Mental Health Costs," 193–200.
213. Herman, *Trauma and Recovery*, 9.

BIBLIOGRAPHY

Adams, George Worthington. *Doctors in Blue: The Medical History of the Union Army in the Civil War*. New York: H. Schuman, 1952.

American Battlefield Trust. "Georgeanna Woolsey: A Day in the Life of a Northern Nurse." www.civilwar.org/learn/articles/georgeanna-woolsey-day-life-northern-nurse.

American Civil War Soldier Letters Home. www.americancivilwar.com/kids_zone/soldiers_letters_civil_war.html.

The American Heritage Dictionary of the English Language. 4th ed. Boston: Houghton Mifflin and Company.

American Psychiatric Association, "Posttraumatic Stress Disorder." 2013. https://www.psychiatry.org/File%20Library/Psychiatrists/Practice/DSM/APA_DSM-5-PTSD.pdf

Aptheker, Herbert. "Negro Casualties in the Civil War." *Journal of Negro History* 32, no. 1 (January 1947): 10–80.

Bacon, Georgeanna Woolsey, and Eliza Woolsy Howland. *Letters of a Family During the War, 1861–65*. Privately published, 1899.

Barton, Brandon. "Cognitive Deficits Are Common in Veterans with Parkinson's Disease." *Neurology Review* 20, no. 8 (August 2014): 32.

Bath VA Medical Center. "VA Medical Center 125th Anniversary Booklet." www.bath.va.gov/docs/125thbooklet.pdf.

Baughman, E. Earl. *Black Americans*. New York: Academic Press, 1971.

Bayne-Jones, Stanhope. *The Evolution of Preventative Medicine in the United States Army, 1607–1939*. Washington, D.C.: Office of the Surgeon General Department of the Army, 1958.

Berlin, Ira. *Free at Last, A Documentary History of the Civil War*. Edison, NJ: Blue and Gray, 1997.

Black, Andrew K. "In the Service of the United States: Comparative Mortality Among African-American and White Troops in the Union Army." *Journal of Negro History* 79, no. 4 (1994): 317–33.

Bollet, Alfred Jay. "An Analysis of the Medical Problems of the Civil War." *Transactions of the American Clinical and Climatological Association* 103 (1992): 128–41.

Brace, Charles, and Emma Brace Donaldson. *The Life of Charles Loring Brace: Chiefly Told in His Own Letters*. New York: C. Scribner's Sons, 1894.

Breslau, N., E.L. Peterson, R.C. Kessler and L.R. Schultz. "Short Screening Scale for DSM-IV Posttraumatic Stress Disorder." *American Journal of Psychiatry* 156, no. 6 (June 1999): 908–11.

Breslau, N., G.C. Davis, P. Andreski and E. Peterson. "Traumatic Events and Posttraumatic Stress Disorder in an Urban Population of Young Adults." *Archives of General Psychiatry* 48, no. 3 (March 1991): 216–22.

Breslau, N., H.D. Chilcoat, R.C. Kessler and G.C. Davis. "Previous Exposure to Trauma and PTSD Effects of Subsequent Trauma: Results from the Detroit Area Survey of Trauma." *American Journal of Psychiatry* 156, no. 6 (June 1999): 902–7.

Bromet, Evelyn. "Risk Factors for DSM-III-R Posttraumatic Stress Disorder Findings from the National Comorbodity Survey." *American Journal of Epidemiology* 147, no. 4 (February 1998): 353–61.

Brown, E. Richard. *Rockefeller Medicine Men: Medicine and Capitalism and America.* Los Angeles: University of California Press, 1981.

Burchard, Peter. *One Gallant Rush: Robert Gould Shaw and His Brave Black Regiment.* New York: St. Martin's Press, 1965.

Burlingame, Michael. *The Inner World of Abraham Lincoln.* Urbana: University of Illinois Press, 1994

Butts, Heather M. *African American Medicine in Washington, D.C.: Healing the Capitol during the Civil War Era.* Charleston, SC: The History Press, 2014.

———. "Alexander Thomas Augusta: Physician, Teacher and Human Rights Activist." *Journal of the National Medical Association* 97, no. 1 (January 2005): 106–9.

Butts, Hugh F. "Black Mask of Humanity." *Journal of the American Academy of Psychiatry and the Law* 30 (2002): 336–39.

Catton, Bruce, and Richard M. Ketchum. *The American Heritage Picture History of the Civil War.* New York, American Heritage Publishing, 1960.

Chadwick, Alex. "Study: Mental Trauma Led to Illness in Civil War Troops." Day to Day, NPR. February 7, 2006. www.npr.org/templates/story/story.php?storyId=5194224.

Civil War Home Page. "Sullivan Ballou's Letter to His Wife." www.civil-war.net/pages/sullivan_ballou.asp.

Clark, Carolyn Chambers. "Posttraumatic Stress Disorder: How to Support Healing," *American Journal of Nursing* 97, no. 8 (August 1997): 26–32.

Cobb, W.M. "Alexander Thomas Augusta, 1825–1890." *Journal of the National Medical Association* 44 (1952): 327–29.

Compas, Bruce E. Jennifer K. Connor-Smith, Heidi Saltzman, Alexandra Harding Thomsen and Martha E. Wadsworth. "Coping with Stress during Childhood and Adolescence: Problems, Progress, and Potential in Theory and Research." *Psychological Bulletin* 127, no. 1 (January 2001): 87–127.

Cook, Kevin. "Dying to Get Home: PTSD in the Civil War." Warfare History Network. December 28, 2018. http://warfarehistorynetwork.com/daily/civil-war/dying-to-get-home-ptsd-in-the-civil-war.

Cordingley, Gary E. and Carl Jon Denbow. "Pioneer African-American Physicians." In *Stories of Medicine in Athens County, Ohio*, ed. Gary E. Cordingley. Baltimore, MD: Gateway Press, 2006.

Crewe, Sandra Edmonds. "Harriet Tubman's Last Work: The Harriet Tubman Home for Aged and Indigent Negroes." *Journal of Gerontological Social Work* 49, no. 3 (2007): 229–44.

Cunningham, H.H. *Doctors in Gray.* Baton Rouge: Louisiana State University Press, 1958.

Deeben, John. "Caring for Veterans in the Nation's Capital." *Prologue* 47, no. 1 (Spring 2015). www.archives.gov/publications/prologue/2015/spring/soldiers-home.html.

de Girolamo, Giovanni, and Alexander Mcfarlane. "The Epidemiology of PTSD: A Comprehensive Review of the International Literature." In *Ethnocultural Aspects of Posttraumatic Stress Disorder: Issues, Research, and Clinical Applications*, edited by A.J. Marsella, M.J. Friedman, E.T. Gerrity and R.M. Scurfield, 33–85. Washington, D.C.: American Psychological Association, 1996.

de Jong, J.T., et al. "Lifetime Events and Posttraumatic Stress Disorder in 4 Post-Conflict Settings." *Journal of the American Medical Association* 286, no. 5 (August 2001): 555–62.

Douglass, Frederick. *Narrative of the Life of Frederick Douglass, An American Slave*. https://docsouth.unc.edu/neh/douglass/douglass.html.

Duncan, Russell, ed. *Blue-Eyed Child of Fortune: The Civil War Letters of Colonel Robert Gould Shaw*. Athens: University of Georgia Press, 1999.

Dyer, Frederick H. *A Compendium of the War of the Rebellion*. Des Moines, IA: Dyer Publishing Company, 1908. www.civil-war.net/searchdyers.asp?searchdyers=Tennessee.

Elliott, Dr. Noah. "African American Pioneer Physician." Wright State University, Annual Conference Presentations, Paper and Posters. April 14, 2007.

Emilio, Luis F. *A Brave Black Regiment: The History of the Fifty-Fourth Regiment of Massachusetts Volunteer Infantry, 1863–1865*. New York: Da Capo Press, 1995.

Evans, Martin C. "Remembering LI Man's Civil War Contribution." Newsday, June 9, 2013. http://www.newsday.com/long-island/remembering-li-man-s-civil-war-contribution-1.5442587.

Faison, Edward Jr. *Racism, the Inevitable in America*. New York: Vantage Press, 1977.

Flannery, Michael. *Civil War Pharmacy: A History of Drugs, Drug Supply and Provision, and Therapeutics for the Union and Confederacy*. London: Informa Healthcare, 2004.

Ford, Sarah. "Suffering in Silence: Psychological Disorders and Soldiers in the American Civil War." *Armstrong Undergraduate Journal of History* 3, no. 2 (April 2013). www.armstrong.edu/history-journal/history-journal-suffering-in-silence-psychological-disorders-and-soldiers-i

Friedman, Matthew J. "History of PTSD in Veterans: Civil War to DSM-5." www.ptsd.va.gov/understand/what/history_ptsd.asp

Fynes, Gene. "Orphanage for Children of Iowa Civil War Soldiers Opened 150 Years Ago on Nov. 16." *Washington Post*, November 16, 2015. www.washingtonpost.com/news/house-divided/wp/2015/11/16/orphanage-for-children-of-iowa-civil-war-soldiers-opened-150-years-ago-on-nov-16.

Garrison, W.B. *Civil War Curiosities: Strange Stories, Oddities, Events, and Coincidences*. Nashville, TN: Rutledge Hill Press, 1994.

Gilder Lehrman Institute of American History. "Donahue, Thomas (fl. 1863) to Almira Winchell." www.gilderlehrman.org/content/almira-winchell-3.

Glatthar, Joseph T. "'Glory,' the 54th Massachusetts Infantry, and Black Soldiers in the Civil War." *History Teacher* 24, no. 4 (August 1991): 475–85.

Gooding, James Henry. *On the Altar of Freedom: A Black Soldier's Civil War Letters from the Front*. Amherst: University of Massachusetts Press, 1991.

Gorrell, Carin. "Noah Wyle and Real Life Trauma," *Psychology Today* (April 2002): 30–34.

Greene, R.E. *African American Defenders of America, 1775–1973*. Chicago: Johnson Publishing, 1974.

Greenhagen, Sue. "Emerson Clark, 92 Last G.A.R Veteran in Putnam, Dies Sunday." SUNY Morrisville. Last modified September 9, 2011. localhistory.morrisville.edu/sites/last_vets/putnamco.html.

Griffiths, D.L. "Medicine and Surgery in the American Civil War." *Proceedings of the Royal Society of Medicine* 59, no. 3 (1966): 204–8.

Haskins, Jim, ed. *Black Stars of Civil War Times*. Hoboken, NJ: John Wiley & Sons, 2002.

Heaver, Stuart. "The Chinese Soldiers Who Fought in the American Civil War." *Post Magazine*, June 30, 2013. www.scmp.com/magazines/post-magazine/article/1270170/gettysburg-redress.

Hendrick, George, and Willene Hendrick. *Black Refugees in Canada: Accounts of Escape during the Era of Slavery*. Jefferson, NC: McFarland, 2010.

Herman, Judith. *Trauma and Recovery*. New York: Basic Books, 1992.

Hildago, Rosario B., and Jonathan R.T. Davidson. "Post Traumatic Stress Disorder Epidemiology and Health Related Considerations." *Journal of Clinical Psychiatry* 61, supplement 7 (2000): 5–13.

Hirsch, E.D. *Cultural Literacy*. 3rd edition. Boston: Houghton Mifflin, 2002.

Holzer, Harold. *Dear Mr. Lincoln: Letters to the President*. Reading, MA: Addison-Wesley, 1993.

Horowitz, Tony. "Did Civil War Soldiers Have PTSD?" *Smithsonian Magazine* (January 2015). www.smithsonianmag.com/history/ptsd-civil-wars-hidden-legacy-180953652.

Humez, Jean M. *The Life and the Life Stories of Harriet Tubman*. Madison: University of Wisconsin Press, 2005.

Jones, Jonathan. "Invisible Wounds: PTSD, the Civil War and Those Who Remained and Suffered." WSKG. February 13, 2016. http://wskg.org/history/invisible-wounds-ptsd-the-civil-war-and-those-who-remained-and-suffered/?c=history.

Karppi, Dagmar Fors. "African American Civil War Museum Honors OB Civil Vet David Carll." *Oyster Bay Enterprise-Pilot*. http://traditionofexcellence.wordpress.com/2010/08/27/african-american-civil-war-museum-honors-ob-civil-war-vet-david-carll.

Kaufman, Howard H. "Treatment of Head Injuries in the American Civil War." *Journal of Neurosurgery* 116, no. 6 (2012): 838–45.

Kessler, R.C. "Posttraumatic Stress Disorder, the Burden to the Individual and to Society." *Journal of Clinical Psychiatry* 61, supplement 5 (2000):4–12.

Kessler, R.C., A. Sonnega, E. Bromet, M. Hughes, C.B. Nelson and N. Breslau. "Epidemiological Risk Factors for Trauma and PTSD." In *Risk Factors for Posttraumatic Stress Disorder*, edited by R. Yehuda, 23–59. Arlington, VA: American Psychiatric Press, 1999.

Klonoff, Elizabeth. "Racial Discrimination and Psychiatric Symptoms Among Blacks." *Cultural Diversity and Ethnic Minority Psychology* 5, no. 4 (November 1999): 320–39. www.researchgate.net/publication/224071379_Racial_Discrimination_and_Psychiatric_Symptoms_among_Blacks.

Korn, Martin. "Emerging Trends in Understanding Posttraumatic Stress Disorder." 154th Annual Meeting of the American Psychiatric Association, May 7, 2001. www.medscape.org/viewarticle/418734.

Lamb, D.S. *A Historical, Biographical and Statistical Souvenir*. Washington, D.C.: Medical Faculty of Howard University, 1900.

Lamberg, Lynne. "Psychiatrists Explore Legacy of Traumatic Stress in Early Life." *Journal of the American Medical Association* 286, no. 5 (August 2001): 523.

Lee, Chulhee. "Socioeconomic Differences in the Health of Black Union Army Soldiers." *Social Science History* 33, no. 4 (2009): 427–57.

Library of Congress. Abraham Lincoln Papers at the Library of Congress. www.loc.gov/collections/abraham-lincoln-papers/about-this-collection.

———. Prints and Photographs Online Catalog (various). http://loc.gov/pictures.

Lively, Matthew. "J.E. Hanger Lost His Leg but Not His Ingenuity." Civil War Profiles. March 16, 2013. http://www.civilwarprofiles.com/category/hanger-james-e.

Lowe, Tony B. "Nineteenth Century Review of Mental Healthcare for African Americans: A Legacy of Service and Policy Barriers." *Journal of Sociology and Social Welfare* 33, no. 4: (2006) 29–50.

MacLean, Maggie. "Annie Haggerty Shaw." Civil War Women. www.civilwarwomenblog.com/annie-haggerty-shaw.

———. "Susan McKinney Steward: First African American Woman Doctor in New York," Civil War Rx. May 16, 2015. http://civilwarrx.blogspot.com/2016/05/susan-mckinney-steward-first-african.html.

Malinenko, Ally. "Susan Smith McKinney Steward: Brooklyn's First Black Woman Physician." Brooklyn Public Library. January 25, 2018. www.bklynlibrary.org/blog/2018/01/25/Susan-smith-mckinney.

Margo, Robert A., and Richard H. Steckel. "The Heights of American Slaves: New Evidence on Slave Nutrition and Health." *Social Science History* 6, no. 4 (1982): 516–38.

Massachusetts Historical Society. Charles E. Briggs letters. www.masshist.org/collection-guides/view/fa0377.

McPherson, James M. *Ordeal by Fire: The Civil War and Reconstruction*, 2nd ed. New York: McGrawHill, 1992.

Meisler, Andrew. "Trauma, PTSD and Substance Abuse." *PTSD Research Quarterly* 7, no. 4 (1996).

Moore, Frank. *The Rebellion Record: A Diary of American Events*. New York: Van Nostrand, 1865.

Morais, Herbert M. *The History of the Afro-American in Medicine*. Cornwells Heights, PA: Publishers Agency, 1978.

Newby, M. Dalyce. *Anderson Ruffin Abbott: First Afro-Canadian Doctor*. Markham, ONT: Associated Medical Services: Fitzhenry & Whiteside, 1998.

Nordenberg, Tamar. "Escaping the Prison of a Past Trauma: New Treatment for Post-Traumatic Stress Disorder." *FDA Consumer* (May–June 2000).

Novae, Andrei. "Traumatic Stress and Human Behavior." *Psychiatric Times* 18 (April 2001).

Oates, Stephen. *A Woman of Valor: Clara Barton and the Civil War*. New York: Free Press, 1994.

O'Brien, Kevin E. *My Life in the Irish Brigade: The Civil War Memoirs of Private William McCarter, 116th Pennsylvania Infantry*. Cambridge, MA: Da Capo Press, 1996.

Operation 300. www.operation300.com.

Osofsky, Joy. "The Effects of Exposure to Violence on Young Children." *American Psychiatrist* 50, no. 2 (September 1995): 782–88.

Painter, Nell Irvin. *Sojourner Truth: A Life, A Symbol*. New York: W.W. Norton, 1997.

Palmer, Sarah Bessie. "The Floating Hospital of St. John's Guild, New York City." *American Journal of Nursing* 4, no. 1 (October 1903).

Pizarro, Judith. "Physical and Mental Health Costs of Traumatic War Experiences among Civil War Veterans." *Archives of General Psychiatry* 63, no. 2 (February 2006): 193–200.

Powers, Bernard Edward. *Black Charlestonians: A Social History, 1822–1885*. Fayetteville: University of Arkansas Press, 1999.

Price, James S. *The Battle of New Market Heights: Freedom Will Be Theirs by the Sword*. Charleston, SC: The History Press, 2011.

Prigerson, "Population Attributable Fractions of Psychiatric Disorders, and Behavioral Outcomes Associated with Combat among US Men." *American Journal of Public Health* 92, no. 1 (2002).

PTSD: General Facts, US Department of Veteran Affairs. www.ptsd.va.gov/understand/what.

PTSD: National Center for PTSD; *PTSD Basics.*www.ptsd.va.gov/understand/what/ptsd_basics.asp.

Quarles, B. *The African American in the Civil War*. New York: Da Capo Press, 1989.

Randolph, Lewis A. *Rights for a Season: Politics of Race, Class, and Gender in Richmond, Virginia*. Knoxville: University of Tennessee Press, 2003.

Reid, Richard M., ed. *Practicing Medicine in a Black Regiment: The Civil War Diary of Burt G. Wilder, 55th Massachusetts*. Amherst: University of Massachusetts Press, 2010.

Rich, John A. "Primary Care for Young African American Men." *Journal of American College Health* 49, no. 4 (2001): 183–86.

Ruthow, Lainie W., and Ira M. Ruthow. "Homeopaths, Surgery and the Civil War: Edward C. Franklin and the Struggle to Achieve Medical Pluralism in the Union Army." *Archives of Surgery* 139, no. 7 (2004): 785–91.

Savitt, T. *Four African-American Proprietary Medical Colleges: 1888–1923*. London: Oxford University Press, 2000.

Schroeder-Lein, Glenna R. *The Encyclopedia of Civil War Medicine*. Armonk, NY: M.E. Sharpe, 2008.

Schultz, Jane E. *Women at the Front: Hospital Workers in Civil War America*. Chapel Hill: University of North Carolina Press, 2004.

Schwartz, Gerald, ed. *A Woman Doctor's Civil War: Esther Hill Hawk's Diary*. Columbia: University of South Carolina Press, 1989.

Scurfield, Raymond Monsour. "Positive and Negative Aspects of Exposure to Racism and Trauma: Research, Assessment and Treatment Implications." *Journal of Ethnic & Cultural Diversity* 10, no. 1 (2001): 23–47.

"Second Annual Report of the Women's Central Association of Relief: No. 10 Cooper Union, New York, May 1, 1863." New York: William S. Dorr, 1863. https://collections. nlm.nih.gov/catalog/nlm:nlmuid-101181516-bk.

Sigaud, Louis A. "When Belle Boyd Wrote Lincoln." *Lincoln Herald*, vol. 50 (February 1948).

Simmons, William J., and Henry McNeal Turner. *Men of Mark: Eminent, Progressive and Rising*. Cleveland, OH: Geo. M. Rewell & Company, 1887.

Soodalter, Ron. "The Shock of War." *America's Civil War Magazine* (May 2017). www.historynet. com/the-shock-of-War.htm.

Steckel, Richard H. "A Peculiar Population: The Nutrition, Health and Mortality of American Slaves from Childhood to Maturity." *Journal of Economic History* 46, no. 3 (1986): 721–41.

Street, James. "Under the Influence: Marching through the Opium Fog." Civil War Rx. http:// civilwarrx.blogspot.com/2014/03/under-influence-marching-through-opium.html.

SUNY Morrisville. "The Civil War Letters of Galutia York." http://localhistory.morrisville. edu/civil_war.

Taylor, Susie King. *Reminiscences of My Life in Camp with the 33rd United States Colored Troops Late 1st S.C. Volunteers*. Boston: self-published, 1902.

Thomson, Samuel. *New Guide to Health, or Botanic Family Physician*. Boston: E.G. House, 1822.

Trimble MR. *Post-traumatic Neurosis: From Railway Spine to the Whiplash*. Chichester, UK: J. Wiley & Sons, 1984.

U.S. Department of Health and Human Services. "Facing Addiction in America: The Surgeon General's Report on Alcohol, Drugs, and Health." 2016. https://addiction. surgeongeneral.gov/sites/default/files/surgeon-generals-report.pdf.

U.S. Department of Veterans Affairs. "PTSD Basics." PTSD: National Center for PTSD. www.ptsd.va.gov/understand/what/ptsd_basics.asp.

———. "PTSD General Facts." www.ptsd.va.gov.

U.S. Senate. "Clara Barton and Senator Henry Wilson." www.senate.gov/artandhistory/ history/common/generic/Civil_War_BartonClara.htm.

van der Kolk, Bessel A. "Assessment and Treatment of Complex PTSD." In *Traumatic Stress*, edited by R. Yehuda. Arlington, VA: American Psychiatric Press, 2001.

Waddell, Joseph Addison. *Annals of Augusta County, Virginia, from 1726 to 1871*, 2nd ed. Staunton, VA: C.R. Caldwell, 1902.

Wikipedia. "31st Infantry Regiment, United States Colored Troops." Last modified August 21, 2018. https://en.wikipedia.org/wiki/31st_Infantry_Regiment,_United_States_Colored_Troops.

Wills, Cheryl. *Die Free*. Minneapolis, MN: Bascom Hill Publishing Group, 2010.

Wilson, Keith P. *Campfires of Freedom: The Camp Life of Black Soldiers during the Civil War*. Kent, OH: Kent State University Press, 2002.

Wilson, Sven E. "Prejudice and Policy: Racial Discrimination in the Union Army Disability Pension System, 1865-1906," *American Journal of Public Health* 100, no. 1 (2010): S56–S65.

Winston, Benjamin. "Smith, Sylvanus." Black Past. www.blackpast.org/aah/sylvanus-smith-1831-1911.

Wooster, Kenneth. "The Diary of Lewis Bramer, Jr." www.Skaneateles.org/lbramer1.html.

Yacovone, Donald, ed. *A Voice of Thunder: The Civil War Letters of George E. Stephens*. Champaign: University of Illinois Press, 1997.

Yale School of Public Health. "Dr. Cortlandt Van Rensselaer Creed: The First African American Graduate of Yale Medical School." Civil War Rx. February 27, 2013. http://civilwarrx.blogspot.com/2013/02/dr-cortlandt-van-rensselaer-creed.html?m=1

Yehuda, Rachel. "Post-Traumatic Stress Disorder." *New England Journal of Medicine* 346, no. 2 (January 2002).

ABOUT THE AUTHOR

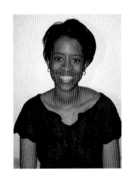 eather Butts, JD, MPH, MA, is an Integration of Science and Practice (ISP) instructor and faculty advisor of the part-time health policy management students at Columbia University Mailman School of Public Health, where she teaches bioethics and public health law. She also serves as an adjunct professor in health law and bioethics at St. John's School of Law. She is the co-founder and a board member of the nonprofit HEALTH for Youths Inc., which focuses on college readiness and preparation. She is also the founder of the online training and education company LEARN for Life Consulting LLC and does college readiness and preparation counseling for high school students.

She previously served as regulatory specialist with Columbia University Medical Center's Institutional Review Board and focused on compliance audits, training, education and privacy issues. Prior to her work at Columbia, Butts served as senior associate in the Healthcare Regulatory Group of Pricewaterhouse Coopers LLP, where she focused on regulatory compliance issues.

Butts received her BA from Princeton University, her JD from St. John's University School of Law, her MPH from Harvard University's T.H. Chan School of Public Health and her MA in education from Columbia University's Teachers College.

Her publications include "Alexander Thomas Augusta: Physician, Teacher and Human Rights Activist."